Trigger Point Therapy for Repetitive Strain Injury

YOUR SELF-TREATMENT WORKBOOK FOR ELBOW, LOWER ARM, WRIST, AND HAND PAIN

Valerie DeLaune, LAc

New Harbinger Publications, Inc.

Distributed in Canada by Raincoast Books

Copyright © 2012 by Valerie DeLaune
New Harbinger Publications, Inc.
5674 Shattuck Avenue
Oakland, CA 94609
www.newharbinger.com

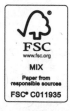

Cover design by Amy Shoup
Acquired by Jess O'Brien
Edited by Jean Blomquist

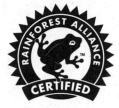

Library of Congress Cataloging-in-Publication Data

DeLaune, Valerie.
  Trigger point therapy for repetitive strain injury : your self-treatment workbook for elbow, lower arm, wrist & hand pain / Valerie DeLaune ; foreword by Renee Gladieux Principe.
     p. cm.
  Summary: "Trigger point expert Valerie DeLaune presents Trigger Point Therapy for Repetitive Strain Injury, a complete treatment manual for healing carpal tunnel syndrome, tennis elbow, and other repetitive strain injuries at home with trigger point therapy"-- Provided by publisher.
  Includes bibliographical references and index.
  ISBN 978-1-60882-127-3 (pbk.) -- ISBN 978-1-60882-128-0 (pdf e-book) -- ISBN 978-1-60882-129-7 (epub)
  1. Overuse injuries--Treatment. 2. Pain--Alternative treatment. 3. Massage therapy. 4. Self-care, Health. I. Title.
  RD97.6.D45 2012
  617.1'72--dc23
                              2011044405

Printed in the United States of America

14   13   12

10   9   8   7   6   5   4   3   2   1

First printing

Contents

Foreword

Renee Gladieux Principe, BA, LMT, NCTMB

Millions of people live with pain every day. For many of these people, the standard medical approach of rest, drugs, and surgery may work. For others, such expensive, conventional care has produced only more pain, depression, and hopelessness.

Perhaps you picked up this book because you are one of those for whom conventional approaches have not worked. If so, what if you learned that the pain you're living with is a direct result of the way you do your job, the way you play, your frenetic lifestyle, or the way you react to stress in your life? What if you discovered that you could relieve your pain yourself? That is what Valerie DeLaune seeks to teach you in this book.

Valerie exemplifies the honorable and crucial tradition of helping those in pain to heal themselves, the greatest gift a healer can give to those who suffer. She contributes greatly to the existing knowledge of myofascial pain due to trigger points. Her lifework involves passing this evidence-based knowledge on to her patients and readers in an understandable and practicable way in order to teach them the self-help techniques that can relieve their pain.

But what does this mean for you, the myofascial pain patient? Valerie's analysis of trigger points reveals that trigger point therapy, whether done by a professional or the person experiencing the pain, deserves a place in mainstream medicine as well as in the nation's health awareness. For the repetitive stress injury patient, she confirms that viable, noninvasive, drug-free options do exist. The problem, however, is that too few health practitioners (a) are qualified to treat trigger points, (b) understand trigger point therapy, and (c) have any experience in treating trigger points. Because of this dearth of qualified practitioners, Valerie maintains that educating you about how to treat your own trigger points remains the best option for achieving lasting, long-term relief.

As with all of Valerie's written work, she bases her methods on sound, accepted scientific research. Through her years of clinical experience, she has formed a realistic approach to healing that encourages her patients to actively participate in the process. Her books demystify the healing process for those suffering from myofascial pain and encourage patients to seek that which serves their own healthy, balanced lifestyle. In this book—as well as in her other books—Valerie invites you to become an active participant in your own healing.

It isn't easy, however, to look at yourself and analyze your daily activities to figure out why you hurt. Most of us move through our days on autopilot, not giving more than a moment's concern to how we perform the tasks that are required of us. But over time, performing repetitive movements and reacting to sudden changes cause our bodies to adapt—and often in very negative ways. That's when we find ourselves weak, in pain, or limited in our ability to move. Reading the first several chapters of this book will help you identify the many factors within your control that may contribute to your own unique pain cycle; the later chapters will teach you how to work with the specific trigger points that contribute to your pain as well as to identify the activities that perpetuate your pain.

When you understand your own pain cycle, you can begin to do something about it. But to do something about that pain, you need to know your options. Valerie wants you to know those options—options that frequently are not included in the information your health care professional gives you. She wants you to know that trigger point self-care is literally at your fingertips and that lifestyle changes may be the secret to reaching your goal of pain-free living. She wants you to become knowledgeable enough to have a dialogue with your family doctor about myofascial pain due to trigger points and have him or her rule them out as a source of your pain before prescribing drugs or issuing a referral to a surgeon. She argues that it is only by truly understanding yourself that can you demand more from our health care system.

As I mentioned above, one source of myofascial pain is repetitive movement. Repeated stress on the upper extremities is a reality of modern, everyday life. Valerie breaks your routine down into understandable terms so you can identify what causes or contributes to your pain. She's helped scores of people understand themselves and their pain in the context of their daily lives—in their work, play, and other life responsibilities. Through this book, she'll help you too.

Of course, there is much that we don't know about the human body. But we do know that muscles make us move, and when movement slows or is restricted, myofascial trigger points are involved in some way. As the science of pain management evolves, we learn more about trigger points. This is good news because we all have trigger points, and trigger points can be treated. Not only can they be identified and treated in a clinical setting with injections, dry needling, spray and stretch techniques, and manual pressure, they can also be self-treated using the same type of direct, manual pressure. In fact, the more you self-treat, the faster you heal!

Therein lies the beauty of this book. Valerie identifies all the common syndromes that afflict the upper extremities. She's the Sherlock Holmes of trigger point self-care, helping you to sleuth your symptoms until you locate and erase all the trigger points that could be causing your pain.

Learning about trigger points, however, is challenging. It requires that you think a little differently about your body. Understanding the nature of referred pain is key. Noticing the anatomy of your muscles helps you visualize your movement patterns. Touching your body, perhaps for the first time with educated intent, is a discovery process. As you enter into this exploration, remember that you didn't get here overnight; untangling the knots will likely take some time, ideally a few minutes daily. And finally, remember that as you successfully treat muscle pain, your muscles will change. The pain will go away, or the pain may migrate. If it doesn't, then you may not be treating the right muscle. With Valerie's book, you can easily use the process of elimination to track down your trigger points.

If there is one thought that you gain from reading and following the guidelines in this book, let it be that you are empowered to take the steps necessary to alleviate your pain. You are not powerless—and must not believe that you are. By educating yourself concerning the realities of your pain and its treatment, you gain the power to pursue and experience healing.

Remember, pain isn't normal. It's a sign that something isn't right. This book will help you to understand why you are in pain. It will also teach you what steps you can take not only to control your pain but also hopefully to alleviate it. And that, I'm sure you'll agree, is great news for you—and for all who suffer from myofascial pain.

Acknowledgments

Approximately 38 percent of the human population is in pain at any given time. Although 30 percent of patients seen in a general physician's practice are there due to pain caused by trigger points (Simons 2003), there is still very little emphasis in medical school on muscle pain and trigger points. Thankfully, a few pioneers have worked endlessly to research trigger points, document referral patterns and other symptoms, and bring all of that information to medical practitioners and the general public.

This book would not have been possible without the life work of Dr. Janet Travell and Dr. David Simons, and my neuromuscular therapy instructor, Jeanne Aland, who introduced me to the books written by Doctors Travell and Simons. All three have now passed on, but I know that I and all of my patients are eternally grateful for their hard work and dedication. Their work lives on through the hundreds of thousands of patients who have gotten relief because of their research and willingness to train others.

Dr. Janet Travell

Dr. Travell was born in 1901 and followed in her father's footsteps to become a doctor. She initially specialized in cardiology but soon became interested in pain relief, as had her father. She joined her father's practice, taught at Cornell University Medical College, and pioneered and researched new pain treatments, including trigger point injections. In her private practice, she began treating Senator John F. Kennedy, who at the time was using crutches due to crippling back pain and was almost unable to walk down just a few stairs. This was at a time when television was just beginning to bring images of politicians into the nation's living rooms, and it had become important for presidential candidates to appear physically fit. Being on crutches probably would have cost President Kennedy the election.

Dr. Travell became the first female White House physician, and after President Kennedy died, she stayed on to treat President Johnson. She resigned a year and a half later to return to her

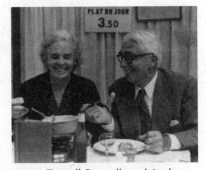

Janet Travell Powell and Jack Powell, 1956. Photo courtesy of Virginia Street.

passions: teaching, lecturing, and writing about chronic myofascial pain. She continued to work into her nineties and died at the age of ninety-five on August 1, 1997.

Dr. David G. Simons

Dr. Simons, who started out his career as an aerospace physician, met Dr. Travell when she lectured at the School of Aerospace Medicine at Brooks Air Force Base in Texas in the 1960s. He soon teamed up with Dr. Travell and began researching the international literature for any references to the treatment of pain. He discovered there were a few others out there who were also discovering trigger points but using different terminology. He studied and documented the physiology of trigger points in both laboratory and clinical settings and tried to find scientific explanations for trigger points. Together Doctors Travell and Simons produced a comprehensive two-volume text on the causes and treatment of trigger points, written for physicians. Dr. Simons continued to research the physiology of trigger points, update the trigger point volumes he coauthored with Dr. Travell, and review trigger point research articles until his death at the age of eighty-seven on April 5, 2010. He was also on the scientific advisory committee of the David G. Simons Academy, which has the goal of internationally promoting the understanding and knowledge of myofascial pain syndrome and trigger point therapy.

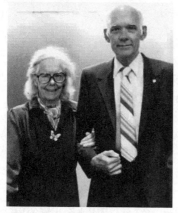

Dr. Janet Travell and Dr. David G. Simons, 1977. Photo courtesy of Dr. David G. Simons.

Other Thanks

Many additional researchers have contributed to the study of trigger points, and many doctors and other practitioners have taken the time to learn about trigger points and give that information to their patients. I would like to acknowledge all of them for their role in alleviating pain by making this important information available.

My editors Jess Beebe, Jess O'Brien, and Jean Blomquist did an excellent job providing organizational suggestions and inspiring me to make each revision even better. I would like to thank David Ham for being the model in the referral pattern photos; and Sarah Olsen for graphic design work. Virginia Street (Janet Travell's daughter) and Dr. Simons provided some of the photos.

I owe many thanks to the thousands of patients and some practitioners who shared with me what worked for them so that I could share that information with you.

Introduction

If you've picked up this book, chances are that you suffer from elbow, lower arm, wrist, or hand pain that occurs frequently or that is intense or debilitating. You need to know that there's seldom a "magic bullet" for curing pain. Until the underlying or perpetuating factors are addressed and the trigger points are treated, pain usually recurs. Upper appendage pain can be an intractable problem because the most common cause is seldom recognized—trigger points in the neck, shoulder girdle, arm, and hand.

What Your Health Care Provider May Not Know

The most important thing to know about trigger points is that they "refer" pain to other areas in fairly consistent patterns. For example, pain felt on the outside of your lower arm may be coming from a muscle in that area (the brachioradialis), but it may also be coming from a trigger point located in a muscle higher up, such as in the front of the neck (the scalenes), underneath the collarbone (the subclavius), or the back or top of the shoulder (the infraspinatus or supraspinatus). Familiarity with referral patterns gives us a starting point of where to look for the trigger points that are actually causing the pain.

Without knowledge of trigger points and referred pain, a health care provider cannot effectively treat pain syndromes. Although trigger points and their referral patterns have been documented for decades and those of us with clinical experience in trigger points have never had any doubt that they are real, only more recently have scientific double-blind controlled placebo experiments been able to "confirm" their existence (Shah et al. 2008; Chen et al. 2007). Though more trigger points studies are being published in scientific and medical journals, word is still slow in getting out to health care providers.

I've treated hundreds of fairly simple cases where people had been told their only recourse was to learn to live with their pain. The reason? Their doctor or other provider didn't know about trigger points or was unwilling to refer to what they may consider an "alternative" practitioner, such as a massage therapist. Thankfully, that's changing. New doctors are exposed to a wider range of alternative treatments in medical school, and some doctors who have practiced medicine for years are getting excited about exploring other treatment options.

I'm frequently contacted by people who are pretty sure trigger point treatment is at least part of the solution to their pain problems, but they are completely frustrated because they can't find a practitioner who knows about trigger points. As of this writing, massage therapists, physical therapists, and physiotherapists are the professionals who are most likely to have experience in treating trigger points. However, even if they do know about trigger points, they may not have learned much about perpetuating factors—the things that cause and keep trigger points activated and that absolutely need to be resolved for long-term relief. This is something I believe is sorely lacking in most trigger point training.

That's why learning about trigger points yourself and doing the self-help exercises in this book is so important; with the information in this book, you may be better equipped to treat trigger points than your health care provider. If you can't find someone who already knows about trigger points, bring this book to your appointments with you. Educate your practitioner about trigger points and your referral patterns. Consumer demand does drive health care, contrary to what a lot of people might think. I've seen this over the past fifteen years with health insurance companies; they are far more likely to cover acupuncture, massage therapy, and manual therapy (such as trigger point therapy, myofascial release, Rolfing, and related types of medical bodywork) than previously, and that's because consumers insisted on it. Health insurance companies are also finally realizing that letting consumers use lower-cost treatments saves them money in the long run.

My Background

I attended massage school in 1989 and learned Swedish massage. I learned to give a very good general massage, but trying to solve a patient's muscular problems was often frustrating and elusive. I saw a class on neuromuscular therapy (which combines a type of deep tissue massage called myofascial release with treating trigger points) in the Heartwood Institute catalog and was intrigued by the description. I attended Jeanne Aland's class in 1991, and it completely changed my approach to treating patients. Once I learned about referral patterns, I was able to start solving problems consistently, even in cases where people had been led to believe they would have to live with their pain.

Over my years of treating thousands of patients, I have added my own observations to those of Doctors Travell and Simons, and have developed a variety of self-help techniques. In 1999,

I received my master's degree in acupuncture. I spent the next twelve years specializing in treating pain syndromes and trigger points with acupuncture. Today I spend most of my time writing about trigger points for both the general public and health care practitioners, in addition to teaching trigger point continuing education classes for providers and teaching self-help classes for the public.

How This Book Is Organized

As you read through this book, you'll learn how muscular problems and repetitive stress injuries in particular can play a very significant role in elbow, lower arm, wrist, or hand pain of any kind. Because trigger points are so often involved in pain, learning self-treatment techniques is critical to obtaining long-term relief.

Part I offers background information on trigger points and why it's important to treat pain as soon as possible, including updates on what's new in trigger point research. The discovery of central sensitization and how it spreads pain to other parts of the body is very important to understanding and treating pain syndromes. Part I also describes the various causes of elbow, lower arm, wrist, and hand pain and their relationship to trigger points.

Part II begins the self-help sections of this book. It will help you identify the factors that are pertinent to your particular set of circumstances and symptoms, and will give suggestions you can take to help resolve them. Many things—including chronic and acute illness, emotional factors, and poor diet—cause trigger points body-wide and keep them activated. Upper appendage pain is most often caused by repetitive stress injuries due to chronically poor posture and ergonomics, and using (and abusing) muscles or muscle groups repetitively. These perpetuating factors will have to be addressed in conjunction with the self-help pressure and stretching techniques in part III in order to resolve your elbow, lower arm, wrist, and hand pain.

Part III provides instructions for locating the muscles that potentially contain trigger points, applying pressure to those trigger points, and stretching the muscles. Chapter 8 describes treatment guidelines in detail, and chapter 9 provides a guide indicating which muscle chapters you will want to consider as potential contributors to your leg, knee, ankle, or foot pain. Chapters 10 through 30 help you identify the specific muscles that are causing your pain. They contain lists of common symptoms for specific trigger points, offer helpful hints for resolving perpetuating factors for those trigger points, and describe self-treatment techniques and stretches.

How to Use This Book

Reading parts I and II will provide you with a foundation for the pressure techniques and stretches that you will learn in part III. Then, as you begin to do the pressure techniques and stretches in part III, you may find it helpful to return to parts I and II. Part II on perpetuating factors may be especially helpful because, in all likelihood, a combination of these perpetuating factors is involved in your pain. You won't get lasting relief from your trigger points (and therefore from your pain) until you address the things that are causing and aggravating your trigger points.

This is not a quick fix! There is no such thing as resolving your chronic pain in fifteen minutes or less or being pain free in five easy steps. No technique or practitioner can do that for you. I recommend that, if possible, you have your trigger points identified by a practitioner who has been trained in treating trigger points, such as a neuromuscular massage therapist or a physical therapist, and use the book to supplement their work. In my experience, people who do self-treatments at home in addition to receiving professional treatments weekly improve at least five times faster than those who receive only professional treatments.

Unfortunately, as I mentioned above, you may not have the option of locating a professional to help you. It could take longer for you to locate trigger points without the guidance of a professional, but with this book, you will most likely be able to locate the trigger points yourself. You will need to read the chapters, search for trigger points in your muscles, and use the self-treatment techniques on a regular basis until your pain is resolved. Ask yourself, "Is it worth some of my time to resolve my pain?" If the answer is yes, then you will find the information in this book very helpful.

Be sure to set realistic goals, otherwise you can get discouraged and give up. It's better to pick just a few things and do them well rather than rush through a greater number of self-help techniques or suggestions and do them poorly. You probably won't be able to apply pressure on five different muscles and stretch them, replace all your office equipment, and change your diet all in the first week. Pace yourself so that this is an enjoyable process, and work on the perpetuating factors over time.

If you're working with a practitioner, they should be able to help you prioritize what needs to be done in the order of importance. If your practitioner is giving you too many things to do at once, be sure to tell them that you are overwhelmed and need to set priorities. Giving a patient too many assignments is all too easy for a practitioner to do, especially when they are first out of school and brimming with many useful ideas and suggestions.

There are hundreds of suggestions in this book. As you read through part II on perpetuating factors and the "Helpful Hints" in chapters about the muscles you have identified as potentially causing your pain referral patterns, highlight anything that might be pertinent to your situation. Then plan to devote some time to accomplishing your goals. Resolving pain is like detective work—what causes your pain and also what resolves it will be a combination of factors unique to you. This book gives you numerous tools for your process of self-discovery on the road to relief from pain.

Part I

TRIGGER POINTS AND ELBOW, LOWER ARM, WRIST, AND HAND PAIN

If you're suffering from elbow, lower arm, wrist, or hand pain, all too often you may be diagnosed with general terms such as repetitive strain (or stress) injury, tennis elbow, golfer's (or thrower's) elbow, tendinitis, carpel tunnel syndrome, thoracic outlet syndrome, pectoralis minor entrapment, or bursitis, without the true cause being identified. Often the cause is trigger points in one or more muscles, but the diagnosing practitioner is unfamiliar with trigger points. Trigger points can play a very large role in most pain syndromes, which means that you may be able to get a great deal of relief, or even complete relief, by working on trigger points and eliminating perpetuating factors.

The sooner you start doing the self-help techniques and possibly receiving treatment from a practitioner, the sooner you will feel better. This is important, since untreated pain can create an escalating cycle that makes it more chronic and more resistant to treatment.

Chapter 1

What Are Trigger Points?

In this chapter, you'll learn what trigger points are, how they form, and what it feels like when they're pressed. You'll also learn how they refer pain to areas of the body remote from the trigger point itself, what symptoms they can cause besides pain, and what happens when they're left untreated.

Characteristics of Trigger Points

Muscle is the largest organ in the human body, typically accounting for almost 50 percent of the body's weight. There are approximately four hundred muscles in the human body (surprisingly, there are individual variations), and any one of them can develop trigger points, potentially causing referred pain and dysfunction. Symptoms can range from intolerable, agonizing pain to painless restriction of movement and distorted posture.

Knots, Tight Bands, and Tenderness in the Muscle

Muscles consist of many muscle cells, or fibers, bundled together and surrounded by connective tissue. Each fiber contains numerous *myofibrils*, and most skeletal muscles contain approximately one thousand to two thousand myofibrils. Each myofibril consists of a chain of sarcomeres connected end-to-end. Muscular contractions take place in the sarcomere.

A *muscle spindle* is a sensory receptor found within the belly of a muscle. Muscle spindles are concentrated where a nerve enters a muscle and also around nerves inside the muscles. Each spindle contains three to twelve *intrafusal muscle fibers*, which detect changes in the length of a muscle. As the body's position changes, information is conveyed to the central nervous system via sensory neurons and is processed in the brain. As needed, the *motor end plate* (a type of nerve ending) releases *acetylcholine*, a neurotransmitter (one of the chemical substances produced and secreted by a neuron and then diffused across *synapses*, or small gaps, between neurons, causing excitation or inhibition of another neuron). The acetylcholine tells the *sarcoplasmic reticulum* (a part of each cell) to release ionized calcium. The *sarcomeres* in the *extrafusal muscle fibers* then contract. When contraction of the muscle fibers is no longer needed, the nerve ending stops releasing acetylcholine, and calcium is pumped back into the sarcoplasmic reticulum. For reasons still not completely known, when a trigger point is present, something stops the muscle fibers from relaxing again. Groups of chronically contracted extrafusal muscle fibers are probably what we feel as a "knot" or "tight band" in the muscle. These muscle fibers are not available for use because they are already contracted, which is why you cannot *condition* (strengthen) a muscle that contains trigger points.

When pressed, trigger points are usually very tender. The sustained contraction of the myofibril leads to the release of sensitizing *neurochemicals* (body substances that affect the nervous system), producing the pain that is felt when the trigger point is pressed. Pain intensity levels can vary depending on the amount of stress placed on the muscles. The intensity of pain can also vary in response to flare-ups of any of the perpetuating factors addressed in part II, including emotional factors, illnesses, and insomnia.

Healthy muscles usually do not contain knots or tight bands, are not tender to pressure, and, when not in use, feel soft and pliable to the touch, not like the hard and dense muscles found in people with chronic pain. People often tell me their muscles feel hard and dense because they work out and do strengthening exercises, but healthy muscles feel soft and pliable when not being used, even if you work out.

Referred Pain

Trigger points may refer pain in the local area and/or to other areas of the body, and the most common patterns have been well documented and diagrammed. These are called *referral patterns*. Trigger points are rarely located in the same place where you feel symptoms. In fact, based on my experience and calculations, body-wide only 26 percent of common trigger points are located within or on the very edge of their *primary area of referral* (the area of referral that is almost always present), approximately 45 percent are located within or on the very edge of their *secondary area of referral* (the area of referral that may or may not be present), and approximately 55 percent are located *remotely* (completely outside either the primary or secondary area of referral). Some of the trigger points included in the 26 percent found in the primary area of referral are less common trigger points in general, or are on the very edge of the area. Sometimes a muscle may contain multiple common trigger points, but only one common trigger point is within the area of primary referral and there are other common trigger points that are either within the secondary pattern or are remote to the pain referral pattern, such as with the trapezius muscle. *Because of this, there is probably realistically only a 14 percent chance of treating a trigger point by working only on the area where you actually feel pain.*

The only trigger points you would actually treat by working on the area in which you feel pain would be in the deltoid in the upper arm; the frontalis in the head; the levator scapula, rhomboids, intercostals, serratus anterior, serratus posterior inferior, and piriformis in the trunk; and the vastus lateralis, gastrocnemius, gracilis, pectineus, plantaris, sartorius, adductor hallucis, and extensors digitorum brevis / hallucis brevis in the leg and foot.

Note that none of the muscles listed are found in the arm. This means that the referred pain in your elbow, lower arm, wrist, or hand will not be treated by working in the area you feel the pain. If you don't search for trigger points remote to where you feel pain, you won't get relief. For example, trigger points in the triceps muscle (the back of your upper arm) can cause pain over the shoulder, the outside of the elbow, the side and back of the lower arm, over the wrist, and sometimes into some of the fingers, in addition to the back of the upper arm (depending on which particular trigger point), and then the pain frequently gets misdiagnosed as tennis elbow, a repetitive strain injury, or carpal tunnel syndrome.

In part III, you'll find guides that help you figure out which muscle chapters to look at initially. Then in each muscle chapter, you will find illustrations of common pain referral patterns that you can compare with your own pain patterns, and this will help you identify the location of the trigger point or points causing your pain.

If you have been in pain for a long time, *central sensitization* (discussed below) can cause the pain referral to deviate from the most commonly found pattern. It may also cause trigger points in several muscles in a region to refer pain to one area, making it all the harder to determine the actual source of the referred pain. This means you can't absolutely rule out the role of a potential trigger point based only on consideration of common referral patterns, since other factors may cause you to have an uncommon referral pattern. The more intense the earlier pain, the more intense the emotions associated with it, and the longer it has gone on, the more likely central sensitization will cause deviation from the most common referral patterns (Simons, Travell, and Simons 1999).

Weakness and Muscle Fatigue

Trigger points cause weakness and loss of coordination of the involved muscles, along with an inability of the muscles to tolerate use. Many people take this as a sign that they need to strengthen the weak muscles, but if the trigger points aren't inactivated first, strengthening (conditioning) exercises will likely encourage the surrounding muscles to do the work instead of the muscle containing the trigger point, further weakening and deconditioning the muscle containing trigger points.

Muscles containing trigger points are fatigued more easily and don't return to a relaxed state as quickly when use of the muscle ceases. In addition, trigger points may cause other muscles to tighten up and become weak and fatigued in the areas where you experience the referred pain, and also cause a generalized tightening of an area as a response to pain.

Other Symptoms

Trigger points can cause symptoms not normally associated with muscular problems. For example, trigger points in the hand and finger extensor muscles, in addition to causing pain in the elbow, lower arm, wrist, and hand, can also cause a weakness of grip that can cause you to drop things unexpectedly or spill while pouring or drinking.

You may suffer from stiff joints, fatigue, generalized weakness, twitching, trembling, and areas of numbness or other odd sensations. It probably wouldn't occur to you (or your health care practitioner) that these symptoms could be caused by a trigger point in a muscle.

Active Phase vs. Latent Phase

A trigger point can be in either an active or a latent phase, depending on how irritated it is. If the trigger point is *active*, it will refer pain or other sensations and limit range of motion. If the trigger point is *latent*, it may cause only a decreased range of motion and weakness, but not pain. The more frequent and intense your pain, the greater the number of active trigger points you're likely to have.

Trigger points that start with some impact to the muscle, such as an injury, are usually active initially. Poor posture or poor body mechanics, repetitive use, a nerve root irritation, or any of the other perpetuating factors addressed in part II can also form active trigger points. Active trigger points may at some point stop referring pain and become latent. However, these latent trigger points can easily become active again, which may lead you to believe you're experiencing a new problem when in fact an old problem—perhaps even something you've forgotten about—is being reaggravated.

Latent trigger points can be reactivated by overuse (including repetitive strain injuries), over-stretching, or muscle chilling. Any of the perpetuating factors discussed in part II can activate previously latent trigger points and make you more prone to developing new trigger points initiated by impacts to muscles. Latent trigger points can also develop gradually without being active first, and you don't even know they are there. In a study of thirteen healthy people with the same eight muscles examined in each (Simons 2003), two people had latent trigger points in seven of those muscles, one person had latent trigger points in six muscles, three had latent trigger points in five muscles, two had latent trigger points in three muscles, two had latent trigger points in two muscles, two had latent trigger points in one muscle, and only one person didn't have latent trigger points in any of the eight muscles! This means that most people have at least some latent trigger points, which can easily be converted to active trigger points. This also means that some people are more prone to developing problems with muscular pain than others.

Primary and Satellite Trigger Points

A *primary*, or *key*, trigger point can cause a *satellite*, or *secondary*, trigger point to develop in a different muscle. The latter may form because it lies within the referral zone of the primary trigger point. Alternatively, the muscle with the satellite trigger point may be overloaded because it's substituting for the muscle that contains the primary trigger point, or it may be countering the tension in the muscle that contains the primary trigger point. When doing self-treatments, be aware that some of your trigger points may be satellite trigger points, in which case you won't be able to treat them effectively until the primary trigger points causing them have been treated. Part III offers guidance in this regard.

Elevated Biochemicals

A groundbreaking 2008 study (Shah et al.) was able to measure eleven elevated biochemicals in and surrounding active trigger points, including inflammatory mediators, neuropeptides, catecholamines, and cytokines (primarily sensitizing substances and immune system biochemicals). In addition, the pH of the samples was strongly acidic compared to other areas of the body. A 1996 study by Issbener, Reeh, and Steen found that a localized acidic pH lowers the pain threshold sensitivity level of sensory receptors (part of the nervous system), even without acute damage to the muscle. This means the more acidic your pH level in a given area, the more easily you will experience pain compared to someone else. Further studies are needed to discover whether body-wide elevations in pH acidity and the substances mentioned above predispose people to develop trigger points.

What Happens When You Leave Trigger Points Untreated?

When people first develop some kind of pain problem, they usually wait to see if it will go away. The problem with "waiting to see" is that when trigger points are left untreated, muscles can be damaged, and eventually changes to the central nervous system can lead to a vicious cycle of pain. This central nervous system involvement probably explains why you are experiencing chronic pain.

Central Nervous System Sensitization

The purpose of the acute stress responses of our bodies is to protect us and let us know we need to change something in our lives, whether it is pulling away from a hot stove burner, fleeing from a dangerous situation, or giving an injured body part time to heal. But when emotional and/or physical stress (including pain) is prolonged, even just for days, there is a maladaptive response: damage to the central nervous system, particularly to the *sympathetic nervous system* and the *hypothalamus-pituitary-adrenal* (HPA) system. This is called central sensitization.

Certain types of nerve receptors in muscles relay information to neurons located within part of the gray matter of the spinal cord and the brain stem. Pain is amplified there and then is relayed to other muscle areas, thereby expanding the region of pain beyond the initially affected area. Once the central nervous system is involved, or *sensitized* in this way, persistent pain leads to long-term or permanent changes in these neurons, which affect adjacent neurons through neurotransmitters. This may also cause the part of the nervous system that would normally counteract pain to malfunction and fail to do its job (Borg-Stein and Simons 2002; Niddam 2009; Latremoliere and Woolf 2009). As a result, pain can be more easily triggered by lower levels of physical and emotional stressors, and also can be more intense and last longer. Conditions of chronic inflammation, such as osteoarthritis and rheumatoid arthritis, also cause central nervous system sensitization, leading to a vicious cycle of pain.

And while prolonged exposure to both emotional and physical stressors can lead to central nervous system sensitization and subsequently cause pain, prolonged pain caused by central nervous system sensitization can lead to emotional and physical stress (Niddam 2009). Just the maladaptive changes in the central nervous system alone can be self-perpetuating and cause pain, even without the presence of either the original or any additional stressors (Latremoliere and Woolf 2009).

So the longer pain goes untreated, the greater the number of neurons that get involved and the more muscles they affect, causing pain in new areas, in turn causing more neurons to get involved—and the bigger the problem becomes, leading to the likelihood that the pain will become a chronic problem. The sooner pain is treated, including addressing the initiating stressors and perpetuating factors, the less likely it will become a permanent problem with widespread muscle involvement and central nervous system changes.

Sensitization of the Opposite Side of the Body

You may be surprised to discover that the same area on the opposite side of your body is also tender to pressure, even though that side isn't otherwise painful. Over half of the time, the opposite side is actually more tender with pressure. Unless it is a recent injury, it's typical for both sides to eventually get involved (for example, if the right calf is painful, there are likely to be trigger points in the left calf). Whatever is affecting one arm is likely affecting the other, whether it's directly from poor body mechanics, poorly designed office furniture, or overuse injuries, or indirectly from chronic degenerative or inflammatory conditions, chronic disease, and central sensitization. For that reason, I almost always work on both sides, and I recommend that you do self-treatments on both sides.

This observation has been supported by a study in which the researchers used needle electrodes placed in the same spot on both sides of the neck or back to record muscle electrical activity (Audette, Wang, and Smith 2004). When an active trigger point was stimulated on one side of the body, it induced electrical muscle activity on the corresponding opposite side. Latent trigger points did not produce the same results. This further supports the concept of central nervous system sensitization, which would cause corresponding trigger points to form on the opposite side of the body over time.

How Trigger Points Form

Trigger points may form after a sudden trauma or injury, or they may develop gradually. Common initiating and perpetuating factors are mechanical stresses, injuries, nutritional problems, emotional factors, sleep problems, acute or chronic infections, organ dysfunction and disease, and other medical conditions. Part II goes into detail about these causes and perpetuators of trigger points.

One of the current theories about the mechanism responsible for the formation of trigger points is the "integrated trigger point hypothesis." If a trauma occurs, or there is a large increase in the motor end plate's release of acetylcholine, an excessive amount of calcium can be released by the sarcoplasmic reticulum. This causes a maximal contracture of a segment of muscle, leading to a maximal demand for energy and impairment of local circulation. If circulation is impaired, the calcium pump doesn't get the fuel and oxygen it needs to pump calcium back into the sarcoplasmic reticulum, so the muscle fiber stays contracted. Sensitizing substances are released, causing pain and stimulation of the *autonomic nervous system* (the part of the nervous system that controls the release of acetylcholine, along with involuntary functions of blood vessels and glands); this results in a positive feedback system with the motor nerve terminal releasing excessive acetylcholine…and so the sarcomere stays contracted. The areas at the ends of the muscle fibers (either at the bone or where the muscle attaches to a tendon) also become tender as the attachments are stressed by the contraction in the center of the fiber (Simons, Travell, and Simons 1999). Once the central nervous system has been sensitized, various substances are released: *histamine* (a compound that causes dilation and permeability of blood vessels), *serotonin* (a neurotransmitter that constricts blood vessels), *bradykinin* (a hormone that dilates peripheral blood vessels and increases small blood vessel permeability), and *substance P* (a compound involved in the regulation of the pain threshold). These substances stimulate the nervous system to release even more acetylcholine locally, adding to the perpetuation of the dysfunctional cycle (Borg-Stein and Simons 2002). This vicious cycle continues until some sort of outside intervention stretches the contracted portion of the muscle fiber. Anxiety and nervous tension also increase autonomic nervous system activity, which commonly aggravates trigger points and their associated symptoms (Simons 2004).

Another current theory is the "muscle spindle hypothesis," which proposes that the main cause of a trigger point is an inflamed muscle spindle (Partanen, Ojala, and Arokoski 2009). Pain receptors activate *skeletofusimotor* units during sustained overload of muscles via a spinal reflex pathway, which connects to the muscle spindles. As pain continues, sustained contraction and fatigue drive the skeletofusimotor units to exhaustion, and cause *rigor* (silent spasm) of the extrafusal muscle fibers, forming the "taut band" we feel as trigger points. Because the muscle spindle itself has a poor blood supply, the inflammatory products of metabolism released will be concentrated products of metabolism inside the spindle and lead to sustained inflammation.

Conclusion

Trigger points are tender when pressed, and the multiple contractures forming the trigger point may feel like a small lump in the muscle. Healthy muscles don't contain trigger points, and they don't feel tender with pressure. If trigger points are left untreated, long-term changes in the central nervous system can lead to a self-perpetuating cycle of trigger points, pain, and muscular damage. Trigger points can cause symptoms other than pain, which should be taken into consideration and may help you determine which muscles contain trigger points. This is particularly important when the referral pattern deviates from the common pattern, making the location of the trigger points harder to determine.

In the next chapter, you'll learn more about treating trigger points and when you should see a doctor.

Chapter 2

You Don't Need to Live with Pain

It is important to treat trigger points as soon as possible so they are less likely to cause chronic pain problems. This chapter explains the importance of prompt treatment, and also gives you some idea of what to expect from treatment and when you might need to consult a health care provider. Part III outlines general guidelines for self-treatment and teaches you how to treat the trigger points involved in elbow, lower arm, wrist, or hand pain.

Pain Is Treatable

People often assume that if a parent had the same type of condition, it must be genetic and they'll just have to learn to live with it. I never operate on the assumption that a condition can't be improved, even if it is genetic. You learn many things from your parents—eating habits, exercise habits, how to deal with stressful situations, even posture and gestures—and all of these things can influence your own health.

I never assume I can't help someone, or that I can't think of someone to refer them to, such as a chiropractor, naturopath, or surgeon who can help them. In spite of being told that you have to learn to live with your medical condition, assume you can change it—at least until you have exhausted all current treatment options.

The Importance of Prompt Treatment

So often I hear patients say, "I kept thinking it would go away." Sometimes symptoms will go away in a few days and never return. But more often, the longer you wait to see if pain will go away, the more muscles become involved in the chain reaction of chronic pain and dysfunction. A muscle hurts and forms trigger points, then the area of referral (where you feel the pain or other symptoms) starts to hurt and tighten up and forms its own satellite trigger points, then those trigger points refer pain somewhere else, and so on. Or the pain may improve for a while, but the trigger points are really just in an inactive phase and can readily become active and cause pain or other symptoms once again.

As explained in chapter 1, eventually there will be sensitization of the central nervous system. The problem gets more complex the longer trigger points are left untreated, becoming more painful, more debilitating, more frustrating, and more time-consuming and expensive to treat. Plus, the longer you wait, the less likely you are to get complete relief—and the more likely it is that your trigger points will be reactivated chronically and periodically.

Breaking the Pain Cycle

Something starts to hurt, so you tense the area up. Then it hurts more, so the muscle tightens up more, perpetuating and escalating the cycle of pain. Any intervention that helps treat trigger points and eliminate perpetuating factors can help break the cycle: trigger point self-treatments, stretching, heat and/or ice, chiropractic or osteopathic treatments, massage, ultrasound, homeopathy, biofeedback, trigger point injections, counseling, and even analgesics.

People are often surprised that I support the use of analgesics, such as aspirin and ibuprofen, but anything that breaks the pain cycle as soon as possible helps prevent the symptoms from getting worse or affecting other muscles. Plus, analgesics can help you tolerate the initial stages of treatment if you are in extreme pain. But be aware that just because your pain level has decreased, this doesn't mean the trigger points are gone. You still need to seek treatment, preferably as soon as possible. Analgesics will most likely take the edge off the pain, but unless you plan to take them as a long-term solution, you also need to treat the source of the problem.

Muscle relaxants are of limited value for people with pain caused by trigger points, because muscle spasms are not the cause of the pain. Also, these drugs first release tension in the muscles that provide *protective splinting* (the muscles that contract to compensate for or protect the weakened muscles containing the trigger points). Removing this protective splinting increases the load on the muscle containing trigger points and leads to additional pain.

Why Trigger Point Therapy Works

Massage and self-treatment of trigger points will allow muscle cells to uptake more oxygen and nutrients and eliminate metabolic wastes again, which is the proper cell metabolism process. Also, pressing on the trigger points and making the muscle hurt a little bit more than it's already hurting causes your body to release pain-masking chemicals such as endorphins, thereby breaking the pain cycle.

How Long Will Therapy Take?

When people begin therapy, they commonly ask me, "How long will it take?" My general rule of thumb is that the longer the condition has been going on and the more medical conditions (of any kind) you have, the greater the number of muscles that will become involved through central sensitization. This means that treatment will be more complex and take longer. If you are perfectly healthy and have only a recent minor injury, you may not need long-term treatment.

Major factors in the amount of time it takes to get relief from symptoms are how diligently you perform self-treatments, and how accurately you identify your perpetuating factors (discussed in part II) and succeed in eliminating them. As I noted in the introduction, in my experience, people who do self-treatments at home in addition to receiving weekly professional treatments improve at least five times faster than those who receive only professional treatments. Doctors Travell and Simons said, "Treatments that are done to the patient should be minimized and effort should be concentrated in teaching what can be done by the patient…. As patients exercise increasing control [over symptom management] they improve both physically and emotionally" (1992, 549).

I can usually give patients a pretty good indication of how many treatments they may need by the end of the second or third treatment, based on their medical condition, how their muscles feel to me, their diligence about self-treatment and working on perpetuating factors, and how much they have improved (or not) within the first few weeks. If you are seeing a practitioner, after a few weeks ask for an assessment of how long and how frequently the practitioner expects to see you. They may be able to at least give you an idea based on what they have seen so far.

A small percentage of people will get worse before they get better, mostly in complex cases. Or the pain may move around, or you may have the perception that the pain moved around only because the worst areas have improved and now you are noticing the next-worst area more. If the self-treatments are uncomfortable, try to find ways to ease the discomfort, such as reducing the frequency of treatments or decreasing the amount of pressure. It's helpful to keep a journal or other record of your pain and other symptoms. Chapter 9 includes a page with a human body outline that you can photocopy and use to document your pain. This will help you determine whether you're making progress, even at times when you don't perceive any changes in your symptoms. Also seek feedback from people who are close to you. Often they will notice progress in your mobility and activity level, even if you aren't aware of it.

I've had only a few cases where I wasn't able to help patients, and in these cases the people were so frustrated (and understandably so) after seeing professional after professional and receiving little or no help that they allowed me to treat them only a few times before giving up, even if they had improved. If you get a little worse before you get better, you may be inclined to give up in the initial stages of treatment. I encourage you to give any treatment you try some amount of time before you decide it isn't working, even if your condition initially gets worse. Most professionals have numerous tools in their bag, and if something isn't working, they can try something else. It is not realistic to expect your practitioner to figure it all out and give you a large amount of relief within the first appointment or two. Just give your practitioner some time to learn your body and observe how you use it. However, if a practitioner doesn't seem to care or have time for you, then by all means look for someone who cares about you getting better.

When Should You See a Health Care Provider?

If you can't get relief by using the self-help techniques in this book, you will need to see a health care provider. It may be that something other than trigger points is causing or contributing to your elbow, lower arm, wrist, or hand pain. X-rays, MRIs, and other diagnostic tests can identify some conditions that may cause pain, such as torn ligaments or tendons, and stress fractures. Referred symptoms due to trigger points can mimic other, more serious conditions or occur concurrently with them. It may take some investigation to determine the ultimate cause of the problem, which will determine how it can most effectively be treated.

You should see a doctor immediately to rule out serious conditions if you have pain in any body part with any of the following symptoms:

- Your pain had a sudden onset, is severe, or starts with a traumatic injury, particularly if you heard a noise at the time.

- Your pain lasts for more than two weeks.

- The intensity of pain increases over time, or the symptoms are different (changes can be an indication of a different, more serious cause).

- Your pain is accompanied by redness, heat, severe swelling, or odd sensations.

- You develop rashes or ulcers that don't heal.

- You are experiencing cramping.

- You develop poor circulation, painful varicose veins, and very cold legs, feet, arms, or hands.

Hopefully your health care provider will rule out any serious conditions. If you are diagnosed with pain from structural damage or chronic conditions, chances are you can relieve much or all of your pain with a combination of self-treatment of trigger points and treating and eliminating the perpetuating factors. Regardless of the diagnosis you receive from a health care provider, my general treatment principle is the same: identify and eliminate all the underlying causes to the extent possible, and treat the trigger points.

Conclusion

The most important thing to learn from this chapter is that you don't necessarily have to live with your pain. There are treatment options, even if your current practitioner isn't aware of all of them. Analgesics, such as ibuprofen, and use of heat and cold can help break the pain cycle, but they are not a substitute for treatment of trigger points and elimination of perpetuating factors. The length of treatment will depend on your individual medical condition and how long the condition has been going on, and your commitment to doing self-treatments and identifying and addressing perpetuating factors. You may possibly get worse before you get better, but this shouldn't necessarily alarm you. If you have any of the symptoms listed above or the self-help techniques in this book aren't helping, see a medical provider.

The next two chapters will address specific types of elbow, lower arm, wrist, or hand pain, and the role of trigger points in causing and perpetuating associated conditions.

Chapter 3

Elbow and Lower Arm Pain

The majority of cases of elbow, lower arm, wrist, and hand pain are caused by repetitive use injuries, whether from hobbies or from work-related or sports-related activities. Traumatic injuries account for a much smaller percentage of chronic upper appendage pain, and an even smaller amount can be accounted for by structural abnormalities. Terms frequently used to describe elbow and lower arm pain are tennis elbow (lateral epicondylitis), golfer's elbow (medial epicondylitis), olecranon bursitis, and thoracic outlet syndrome. These are likely due either all or in part to referred pain and/or tightness caused by trigger points. Even if pain was initiated by a traumatic injury, trigger points were likely formed as a result of the injury, and will need to be treated for lasting relief.

Tennis Elbow/Lateral Epicondylitis

Pain on the outside bony prominence of the elbow (*epicondyle*) is usually labeled "tennis elbow," and is also known as *lateral epicondylitis*. This condition originally got its name because onset was most often caused by playing tennis and was thought to be caused by inflammation of a tendon. Computer use is more likely the culprit in the vast majority of cases in recent decades. Most current medical literature, unfortunately, has still not recognized the role of trigger points, even though it is now acknowledged that inflammation of the tendon is uncommon. The signs, symptoms, and causes of "lateral epicondylitis" are identical to those of trigger points in the associated muscles on either side of the joint.

Trigger points that cause pain in the area of the lateral epicondyle are likely to develop in the following order: supinator (chapter 25); brachioradialis (chapter 24); extensor carpi radialis longus (chapter 24); extensor digitorum (chapter 24); triceps (chapter 19); anconeus (chapter 19); and the biceps brachii (chapter 23) and brachialis (chapter 28) together. Check the muscle chapters cited in parentheses for self-help techniques, and you will likely be able to resolve your lateral epicondylitis.

Golfer's (or Thrower's) Elbow/Medial Epicondylitis

Pain on the inside bony prominence of the elbow is usually labeled golfer's or thrower's elbow, and is also known as *medial epicondylitis*. As with lateral epicondylitis, most current medical literature has still not recognized the role of trigger points.

Pain referred to the medial epicondyle may be caused by trigger points in the triceps brachii (chapter 19), pectoralis major (chapter 11), pectoralis minor (chapter 21), serratus anterior (chapter 12), and serratus posterior superior (chapter 15). You will also want to check for trigger points in all of the hand and finger flexors (chapter 27) and extensors (chapter 24), in case tightness in those muscles are contributing to your pain.

Olecranon Bursitis

If there is pain combined with swelling on the pointy part of the elbow (the *olecranon process*), it is more likely due to inflammation within the fluid-filled sac called a *bursa*. This condition can be caused either by an impact injury or by repetitively leaning on your elbow against a hard surface, such as a desk. If swelling was caused by an impact injury, it will likely be a larger (and hence more noticeable) area of swelling than that caused by a repetitive injury, and could be due to a triceps rupture. If you have swelling around the olecranon process, do not lean on your elbows (which in any case is poor ergonomics!), and try applying an ice pack. Acupuncture and Traumeel ointment (a homeopathic ointment with arnica and other ingredients) will likely be helpful. You may need to see a health care provider who can rule out a triceps rupture or remove the excess fluid from the bursa with a needle.

Trigger points in the triceps and/or serratus posterior superior will also refer pain to the olecranon process, but without accompanying swelling. Keep in mind that trigger points may occur concurrently with olecranon bursitis, and they will almost certainly form as a result of any kind of impact or repetitive use injury. Trigger points and/or tightness in the triceps brachii muscle will predispose the muscle to sustaining an injury.

Thoracic Outlet Syndrome

Thoracic outlet syndrome (TOS) is a collection of symptoms rather than a specific disease, though health care providers often use the term as though it were a particular condition. There is widespread disagreement and confusion in most medical literature about what symptoms define the condition and what causes it. TOS pain may be felt in the neck, shoulder, forearm, and hand, and may be accompanied by numbness, tingling, and weakness. Trigger points are frequently overlooked as a cause of abnormal tension in the scalene muscles, and are most likely a major cause of thoracic outlet syndrome, though it might more aptly be called *pseudo–thoracic outlet syndrome.*

Travell and Simons (1999, chapter 20, "Scalene Muscle") provide a lengthy discussion of the use of the term "thoracic outlet syndrome," and if your health care provider has used this diagnosis, I highly recommend that you read the chapter and share the information with them. It is definitely worth having a trained practitioner check all of the muscles listed in the next paragraphs to see if you may be harboring trigger points, especially if you are considering surgery. Surgery has a less than 50 percent success rate for thoracic outlet syndrome, most likely because trigger points haven't been considered or relieved. Additional problems often develop subsequent to the unsuccessful surgeries. There may be a few patients with anatomical abnormalities that require surgical correction for complete relief, but the majority of patients will have a higher success rate with non-surgical intervention.

Trigger points in the scalenes (chapter 20), pectoralis major (chapter 11), latissimus dorsi (chapter 17), teres major (chapter 18), and subscapularis (chapter 16) muscles can all refer pain in patterns that mimic thoracic outlet syndrome symptoms, and it can be particularly confusing if more than one muscle develops trigger points. Trapezius (chapter 10) and pectoralis minor (chapter 21) trigger points can also refer pain that might get diagnosed as thoracic outlet syndrome. Be sure to check *all* of those muscles. The subclavius muscle (chapter 11) can become enlarged and may cause the first rib to be elevated and compress the subclavian vein, so check for trigger points in that muscle too, and see a chiropractor or osteopathic physician to determine if the first rib needs to be adjusted.

Also check the supraspinatus (chapter 13) and infraspinatus (chapter 14) muscles for associated trigger points. Satellite trigger points tend to develop in the triceps brachii (chapter 19), pectoralis major and minor (chapters 11 and 21), and hand extensor (chapter 24) muscles. Trigger points in the levator scapula may also refer pain that might get diagnosed as TOS, the sternocleidomastoid and splenius capitis may also contain associated trigger points, and the deltoid may also develop satellite trigger points, but because trigger points in these muscles don't directly cause elbow, lower arm, wrist, and hand pain, they are not addressed in this book. See the Resources section for additional trigger point books that include these muscles.

Elbow Injuries

If your elbow is suddenly bent the wrong way (hyperextension), it can damage the ligaments and other structures in and around the joint. If the force of an injury is great enough (probably from a fall or direct blow), the elbow joint can be dislocated, and it will usually be accompanied by a fracture of one or more of the bones in the upper or lower arm: the humerus (upper arm), ulna, or radius (lower arm). A medial elbow collateral ligament sprain can also be caused by repetitive motions that are fairly vigorous (such as repetitively throwing something heavy).

If you have had either a traumatic or repetitive use injury that has caused one or more of these problems, trigger points have likely formed and should be treated to prevent chronic pain. Also, some of the bones may have been misaligned, and they should be adjusted by a chiropractor or osteopathic physician.

Conclusion

Trigger points are most likely involved in any kind of elbow and/or lower arm pain, whether they are the source of the pain or were formed subsequent to injury. See the pain guides in chapter 9 to determine which muscles to check for trigger points, based on the location(s) where you feel your symptoms. Trigger points may also cause numbness and tingling, so check *all* areas where you feel symptoms, and not just where you feel pain.

With any shoulder, upper arm, or elbow problems, you may find it helpful to lie in one of the positions shown in these photos to reduce pain and other symptoms at night, in addition to applying pressure and stretches for individual muscles and related trigger points.

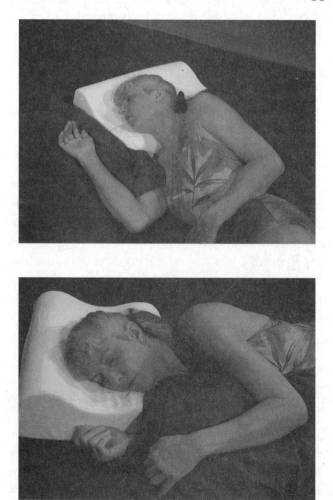

Chapter 4

Wrist, Hand, and Finger Pain

Unless wrist, hand, or finger pain has been caused by a traumatic injury, the symptoms are more likely the result of a *repetitive strain injury*—a general term used to describe pain brought on by repetitive overuse movements, whether work, hobby, or sports related.

The use of computers has caused a huge increase in the number of patients with referred pain from trigger points in the forearm muscles. Often patients will complain of pain in the wrist and/or hand, and subsequently may have been misdiagnosed with *carpal tunnel syndrome*. They are often given a brace to wear, which may afford some relief but does not solve a trigger point–caused problem.

Other, less common conditions that cause wrist, hand, or finger pain or other symptoms are wrist bursitis, de Quervain's tenosynovitis, trigger finger/thumb, Dupuytren's contracture, and Heberden's nodes. Treating trigger points and associated muscle tightness will likely help resolve these conditions, or at least minimize the accompanying pain.

Repetitive Strain Injury (RSI)

Repetitive overuse, resulting in the formation of trigger points, accounts for the majority of cases of onset of upper appendage pain and other symptoms. Therefore, treatment of trigger points can resolve most cases of arm, elbow, wrist, hand, and finger pain. As with the conditions discussed in chapter 3, most current medical literature has still not recognized the role of trigger points. The signs, symptoms, and causes of repetitive strain injury are identical to those of trigger points in the associated muscles.

Carpal Tunnel Syndrome

Carpel tunnel syndrome may occur in conjunction with thoracic outlet syndrome (see chapter 3), or the symptoms of carpal tunnel syndrome may be mimicked by trigger points, in which case the condition is more aptly called *pseudo-carpal tunnel syndrome*. The carpal tunnel consists of the transverse carpal ligament located on the palm side of the hand just below the wrist, and the eight wrist bones that form the other three sides of the tunnel. When one of the nine long flexor tendons passing through the tunnel swells or degenerates, or something causes the tunnel to get smaller, the narrowing of the canal can result in compression or entrapment of the median nerve. This causes burning, numbness, tingling, weakness, or muscle damage in the hand and fingers.

True carpal tunnel syndrome is likely caused by using tools that vibrate or by prior injuries, such as a broken or sprained wrist that caused swelling. Some people have a smaller carpal tunnel and are more predisposed to having problems as a result. There are several predisposing systemic factors that may play a part, such as an overactive pituitary gland, hypothyroidism, rheumatoid arthritis, or fluid retention during pregnancy or menopause.

The majority of carpal tunnel syndrome diagnoses are in fact *mis*diagnoses and are really symptoms caused by trigger points. If you have been diagnosed with carpel tunnel syndrome, it's worth checking for trigger points in the scalenes (chapter 20), pectoralis minor (chapter 21), biceps (chapter 23), brachialis (chapter 28), coracobrachialis (chapter 22), hand and finger extensors and brachioradialis (chapter 24), hand and finger flexors / pronator teres (chapter 27), palmaris longus (chapter 26), and adductor/opponens pollicis (chapter 29).

A *pectoralis minor entrapment*, where the pectoralis minor muscle is chronically tight from trigger points or other causes and its tendon pinches the axillary artery and the brachial plexus nerve, can be misdiagnosed as carpal tunnel syndrome and will not be resolved by surgery on the carpal tunnel. Entrapment of the brachial plexus nerve causes numbness and uncomfortable sensations in the ring and little fingers, back of the hand, outside of the forearm, and palm side of the thumb, index, and middle fingers. Check the pectoralis minor (chapter 21) and also the biceps (chapter 23), coracobrachialis (chapter 22), and trapezius (chapter 10) muscles for associated trigger points.

If you are considering surgery, be sure to treat the trigger points yourself and, ideally, get the assistance of a trained practitioner to ensure your success. Surgery has a poor rate of success, likely due to referred symptoms from trigger points not being considered as the cause.

Wrist Bursitis

The fluid-filled lubricating sac called a bursa, which in the case of the wrist extends over part of the back of the hand and a short distance up the lower arm, becomes inflamed and swollen. The most common causes are sports-related activities such as baseball, badminton, tennis, and cycling, but repetitive strain injuries of any kind can cause wrist bursitis to develop. Symptoms include a lump or swelling on the back side of the wrist and pain that is worse when you put weight on your hand with the wrist bent backwards, as with bicycling. Try applying ice to the area and avoid or minimize aggravating activities. Treat any trigger points in the arm and hand. Acupuncture and Traumeel ointment will likely be helpful. You may need to see a health care provider who can remove the excess fluid from the bursa with a needle.

Sprains and Fractures

The thumb can easily be sprained by being bent backward, and is usually caused by falling with an outstretched hand, or during sports activities, including skiing, basketball, and any kind of contact sport. Fractures of the bones of the lower arm (radius or ulna), wrist bones, and/or finger bones can also occur for the same reasons. You may need to get an X-ray for diagnosis, or possibly an MRI. Ice, rest, and/or immobilization may be necessary. Arnica, Traumeel, and/or Chinese herbs for pain and trauma will be helpful. Trigger points will form as a result of any kind of injury, so after swelling is reduced and/or a cast is removed, begin to gently treat your trigger points.

De Quervain's Tenosynovitis

De Quervain's tenosynovitis (also known as de Quervain's disease or syndrome) is an inflammation of the connective tissue sheath surrounding the pronator teres (chapter 27) and abductor pollicis longus muscles where they cross the thumb side of the wrist. It is commonly initiated by a blow to the thumb, by any repetitive grasping such as with gardening, or by sports activities such as racquet sports, canoeing, bowling, or golfing. Inflammatory diseases such as rheumatoid arthritis can also trigger tenosynovitis. Pain alone should not be used to make a positive diagnosis, since trigger points will be initiated and aggravated by the same activities. If you have swelling over the wrist on the thumb side, you may have de Quervain's tenosynovitis. Try applying ice, and treating trigger points in the forearm (chapters 24, 25, 27, and 28) and thumb (chapter 29).

Trigger Finger and Trigger Thumb

Trigger finger, where the finger gets "stuck" in the fist-closed position, is caused by a constriction of a tendon in the palm, about one-thumb's width above the crease between the palm and the finger. *Trigger thumb*, where the thumb locks in the closed position, can be caused by a tender spot in or near one of the forearm flexor tendons located under the thumb pad or in the web between the thumb and first finger. The cause of trigger finger is unclear, but may possibly be caused by pressing something relatively pointy repeatedly into the palm. See the chapters on hand and finger flexors (27), and adductor/opponens pollicis (29) for self-help treatments that may help resolve trigger finger and trigger thumb, even though trigger points aren't directly responsible.

Dupuytren's Contracture

Dupuytren's contracture is a condition where the connective tissue in the palm becomes fibrous and thickened, subsequently contracting and causing the fingers to curl. The ring and little fingers are affected most often, and the middle finger may become involved as the condition slowly progresses. It rarely affects the index finger and thumb. Nodules form in the palm adjacent to the affected fingers, and they are initially tender. In advanced cases of Dupuytren's contracture, the palm is contracted and you can't lay your hand flat on a surface, but pain tends to decrease over time. Dupuytren's contracture is more common in men and in people with alcoholism, diabetes, and epilepsy, and tends to develop mostly in midlife, generally when people are in their late thirties, their forties, or their early fifties.

Tightness and trigger points in the palmaris longus muscle, because of its action on cutaneous tissue in the palm, are factors in the development of the nodules and fibrous bands. Performing the self-help techniques on the palmaris longus muscle (chapter 26) can possibly stop the progression of nodule formation. Also try working on the hand and finger flexors (chapter 27). Acupuncture may also help; plum blossom technique over the nodules and needles inserted into the palmaris longus and other hand and finger flexors have been successful.

Current surgical guidelines are that if you can still lay the hand flat, no treatment is given. If the condition has progressed to the point that it is interfering with your activities, then consult with a surgeon.

Heberden's Nodes

Heberden's nodes are hard bumps about the size of a pea found on one side of the joint closest to the fingertip. They are initially tender, but pain usually decreases over time. Heberden's nodes are more common in women, and often form within three years after menopause.

If you have Heberden's nodes, look for trigger points in the interosseous muscles (chapter 30), since they may be an initiating factor. Once the trigger points are inactivated, tenderness should disappear immediately, and over time the node itself will probably disappear.

Conclusion

Trigger points are most likely involved in any kind of wrist and/or hand pain, whether they are the source of the pain or were formed subsequent to injury. See the pain guides in chapter 9 to determine which muscles to check for trigger points, based on the location(s) where you feel your symptoms. Trigger points may also cause numbness and tingling, so check *all* areas where you feel symptoms, and not just where you feel pain.

Part II

WHAT CAUSES TRIGGER POINTS AND KEEPS THEM GOING: PERPETUATING FACTORS

According to Doctors Janet Travell and David G. Simons (1983), "If we treat myofascial pain syndromes without…correcting the multiple perpetuating factors, the patient is doomed to endless cycles of treatment and relapse…. Usually, one stress activates the [trigger point], then other factors perpetuate it. In some patients, these perpetuating factors are so important that their elimination results in complete relief of the pain without any local treatment" (103).

This section outlines some general causes that activate or perpetuate trigger points and offers many suggestions on how to address the perpetuating factors to help you eliminate elbow, lower arm, wrist, or hand pain. (In part III, the chapters on individual muscles will give you additional suggestions specific to each muscle.) I recommend you read each chapter to learn how body mechanics, diet, and other perpetuating factors may contribute to your pain. Multiple factors are often involved, and up to this point, you may not have been aware that these factors could be contributing to your pain. Common perpetuating factors include mechanical stressors, injuries, spinal misalignments, nutrient deficiencies, poor dietary habits, food allergies, emotional factors, sleep problems, acute or chronic infections, hormonal imbalances, and organ dysfunction and disease.

As you address perpetuating factors, pace yourself so that the process isn't too overwhelming. Work on your perpetuating factors over time. You probably can't make all the needed changes at once. As you begin to address your perpetuating factors, go ahead and start on the self-help techniques in part III. Applying pressure to trigger points will probably relieve pain and other symptoms either temporarily or for the long term; however, it won't resolve the underlying perpetuating factors. If you get temporary relief from trigger point therapy but your symptoms quickly recur, then trigger points are definitely a factor, but you'll need to address perpetuating factors to gain more lasting relief.

Chapter 5

Body Mechanics

How you sit, stand, walk, run, move, and generally treat your muscles has a great influence on whether or not you form or perpetuate trigger points. In the case of elbow, lower arm, wrist, or hand, paying particular attention to posture, ergonomics, and how you use your muscles will greatly speed your healing and help provide long-term relief. Even learning proper head positioning is critical to treating trigger points, since head-forward posture can cause and perpetuate trigger points that can refer pain all the way down into your fingers. Treating new injuries promptly can help prevent the formation of trigger points, and the treatment of older injuries, as well as spinal misalignments and other problems in the skeletal system, can help stop the perpetuation of trigger points.

Mechanical Stressors

Chronic mechanical stressors such as sitting in poorly designed chairs and at poorly designed workstations, playing sports without proper warm-up, and skeletal asymmetries will cause a self-perpetuating cycle of trigger point aggravation. They are among the most common causes and perpetuators of trigger points involved in elbow, lower arm, wrist, or hand pain. Fortunately most are nearly always correctable, and minimizing or eliminating them is one of the most important things you can do to break your cycle of pain.

Abuse of Muscles

Playing sports can cause trigger points due to a number of factors: improper warm-up, overusing certain muscles or muscle groups while underusing others, receiving direct blows to body parts, experiencing strains and sprains, tendon ruptures, and fractures. You are particularly susceptible if you are a "weekend warrior" and do strenuous athletic activities only a day or two per week.

Your posture can affect your entire body. If you slouch at your desk or on your couch, or if you read in bed, your muscles will suffer, all the way down into your hands and fingers, legs, and feet. Abuse of muscles includes poor body mechanics (such as lifting improperly), long periods of immobility (such as sitting at a desk or standing without a break), repetitive movements (such as scooting your chair around using your legs), and holding your body in awkward positions for long periods, such as squatting. The self-help techniques listed below will help you prevent abuse of your muscles.

Self-help technique: Train and warm up properly for sports. Stretch adequately before each activity, cross-train so you build up all muscles, and increase repetitions and weights gradually to reduce risk of injury.

Self-help technique: Take frequent breaks. Anytime you must sit or stand for long periods, take frequent breaks. One good trick is to set a timer across the room; you'll have to get up to turn it off. Vary your activities so you are not doing any one thing for very long, particularly anything involving repetitive movements that use your shoulders, forearms, or hands.

Self-help technique: Be aware of your body mechanics. Be sure to sit straight with your back against a proper support (discussed below). Learn to lift properly using your knees, not your back.

Misfitting Furniture

Misfitting furniture is a major cause of muscular pain, particularly in the workplace, and specifically for repetitive strain injuries. Sitting at a desk or computer, whether at work or home, places a great deal of stress on your muscles, which can affect your entire body. But there are many things you can do to improve your office setup, and many of them aren't too expensive, such as lumbar supports, phone headsets, and copyholders. Just sticking a thick catalog under your computer screen to raise it to the proper height can make a big difference. Having these gadgets readily available will ensure you use them as much as possible.

Get Office Furniture That Fits You

Modifying or replacing misfitting furniture is one of the easiest things you can do to help get relief from trigger points, particularly those affecting your arm and hand. Once it's done, you won't have to do it on a daily or frequent basis as part of your self-help. You'll still need to be aware of your posture, but furniture that corrects some of your counterproductive postural habits without you having to be aware of them is much simpler. Consider contacting a company that specializes in ergonomics to come to your workplace and assess your office arrangement. They can make some adjustments and help you select furniture that fits your body. Your employer may balk at the cost, but if you end up with health problems as a result of a poor workstation, they'll end up paying for it in lost work time and workers' compensation claims. If your employer won't pay for this, consider paying for it yourself. What is it worth to you to be pain free?

Chair. Your elbows and forearms should rest evenly either on your work surface or on armrests of the proper height. The armrests must be high enough to support your elbows without you leaning to the side, but not so high as to cause your shoulders to hike up. The upholstery needs to be firm. Your knees should fit under your desk, and your chair needs to be close enough that you can lean against your backrest. A good chair supports both your lumbar area and your mid-back. The seat should be low enough that your feet rest flat on the floor without compression of your thighs by the front edge of the seat, high enough that not all the pressure is placed on your gluteal area, and slightly hollowed out to accommodate your buttocks. If you cannot sit at the proper height for your desk and computer as well as rest your feet on the floor, you may need to get a footstool in order to avoid compression of your hamstring muscles. If you look around, you can get a good adjustable chair for around $120.

Computer screen. Your computer screen should be directly in front of you, slightly below eye level and slightly tilted back at the top. If you work from hard copy, attach it to the side of the screen with a copyholder so that you can look directly forward as much as possible rather than tipping your head down or turning it too far to the side. You can raise the height of your screen by placing catalogs or books underneath it until it's at the correct level. Evaluate your workstation to make sure that you don't have glare on your screen, that the screen isn't bothering your eyes, and that your lighting is adequate.

Keyboard and mouse. If you have a keyboard tray, it should be height-adjustable. Your forearms should be parallel to the floor, and your wrists should be straight. You may want to use a wrist rest. I see a lot of what I call "mouse injuries," that is, arm and shoulder pain due to using a computer mouse for extended periods without proper arm support.

Headset. A telephone headset can provide a great deal of relief from neck and back pain, which can affect you all the way into your arms and hands. Telephone shoulder rests aren't adequate, and if you try to hold the phone in your hand, you'll end up cradling it between your head and shoulder at some point, which is very hard on your neck and trapezius muscles. Get headsets for all of your phones—at work, at home, and for your cell phone.

Lumbar support. A lumbar support helps correct round-shouldered posture. Most chiropractic offices carry lumbar supports of varying thickness. I recommend that you get one for your car and one for your favorite seat at home. Try to avoid sitting on anything without back support, since this causes you to sit with your shoulders and upper back slumped forward. When going to sporting events, picnics, or other places where you won't have back support, bring a Crazy Creek–brand chair or something similar to provide at least some support. You can get one through most major sporting goods suppliers. They cost only about forty dollars—a good investment in your back—and they're very lightweight for carrying. Or consider a lightweight collapsible chair, also available at sporting goods stores.

Bedtime Furniture

You probably spend about one-third of your time in bed, so it is extremely important to make sure your pillows and bed are right for you. Sleeping on a couch or in a chair should definitely be avoided.

Pillows. If your pillow is made from foam rubber or some other springy material that will jiggle your neck, get rid of it! Vibrations from these pillows will aggravate trigger points in the back and neck, which can subsequently affect the shoulders, arms, and hands. (However, memory foam pillows are fine.) Your pillow should support your head at a level that keeps your spine in alignment and is comfortable when you are lying on your side. Chiropractic offices usually carry well-designed pillows. I always take my pillow with me when I travel; that way I know I have something comfortable to sleep on, and it comes in handy if I get stuck in an airport.

Bed. A bed that is too soft can cause a lot of muscular problems, even in your arms and hands. You may not even realize that your bed is too soft. People usually insist their mattress is firm enough, but when queried further they admit that sleeping on a mat on the floor gives them relief when their pain is particularly bad. Try putting a camping mat on the floor and sleeping on it for a week. If you feel better, your mattress isn't firm enough, no matter how much money you spent on it or how well it worked for someone else. Different people need different kinds of mattresses. An all-cotton futon is very firm and may be best for some people. Mattresses really last only about five to seven years, and after that time they should be replaced. Also consider that if your partner is heavier, you may be unaware that you brace yourself slightly in order not to roll into him or her. Some types of mattresses can accommodate couples who need different degrees of firmness.

Clothing

You may be surprised to learn that what you wear and how you wear it can cause or perpetuate trigger points. Since constricting clothing can impair circulation, it can directly cause trigger points. Fortunately clothing is a problem that's easily correctable, as you will see in the self-help techniques below.

Self-help technique: Choose appropriate footwear and get orthotics. Don't wear high heels, cowboy boots, or other shoes with heels.

While correcting foot supination (more weight on the outside of your foot) or pronation (more weight on the inside of your foot) is essential for some people, almost everyone can benefit from using some kind of foot support inserted in their shoes. Shoes rarely have adequate arch support, and this affects muscles all the way up through your body. My favorite noncorrective orthotics are the Superfeet brand. They have a deep heel cup, which helps prevent pronation and supination, and they provide excellent arch support. Superfeet has a variety of models, including cheaper, noncustom trim-to-fit insoles and moderately priced custom-molded insoles. Their products can provide support in a wide variety of footwear. Visit superfeet.com to learn more about their products. If you find you need corrective orthotics, you will need to see a podiatrist.

Self-help technique: Loosen your clothing. Constricting clothing can lead to impaired circulation and muscular problems. My rule of thumb is if clothing leaves an elastic mark or indentation on your skin, it is too tight and is cutting off proper circulation. Check your socks, belts, waistbands, bras, and ties to see if they're too tight. Tight bras and neckties in particular can cause and perpetuate trigger points in the arms and hands.

Self-help technique: Carry your purse or daypack properly. If you carry a purse, get one with a long strap and put the strap over your head so you wear it diagonally across your torso rather than over one shoulder, and keep its contents light. If you use a daypack, put the straps over both shoulders. When you carry a purse or pack over one shoulder, you have to hike up that shoulder at least a little to keep the strap from slipping off, no matter how light your purse or pack may be. When you are hiking up one shoulder, you are affecting muscles all the way down the arm.

Head-Forward Posture

Head-forward posture leads to the development and perpetuation of trigger points throughout the entire body, but will particularly affect the scalene muscles. The scalenes frequently harbor trigger points responsible for arm and hand pain, which leads to frequent misdiagnosis of carpal tunnel syndrome and thoracic outlet syndrome. If you are not sure whether you chronically hold your head forward, stand in a position that is normal for you, and have someone look at your side profile to see if your head is farther forward than your trunk. The farther you hold your head forward of your shoulders, the more trigger points you're likely to develop (Marcus et al. 1999). Postural exercises can help eliminate head-forward posture.

Self-help technique: Use lumbar support. Poor posture while sitting—whether in a car, at a desk, in front of a computer, or while eating dinner or watching TV—can cause or aggravate head-forward posture. Using a good lumbar support everywhere you sit will help correct poor sitting posture and, ultimately, head-forward posture.

Self-help technique: Do postural exercises. To develop proper posture and reduce head-forward posture, stand with your feet about four inches apart, with your arms at your sides and your thumbs pointing forward. Tighten your buttocks to stabilize your lower back, and then, while inhaling, rotate your arms and shoulders out and back (rotating your thumbs backward) and squeeze your shoulder blades closer together behind you. While holding this position, drop your shoulders down and exhale. Move your head back to bring your ears in line with your shoulders, and hold this position for about six seconds while breathing normally. (When moving your head, don't tilt your head up or down or open your mouth.) Relax, but try to maintain good posture once you release the pose. If holding this position feels uncomfortable or stiff, try shifting your weight from your heels to the balls of your feet, which will cause your head to move backward over your shoulders. Repeat this exercise frequently throughout the day to develop good posture. Do it every hour or two. It is better to do one repetition six or more times per day than to do six repetitions in a row (Travell and Simons 1983).

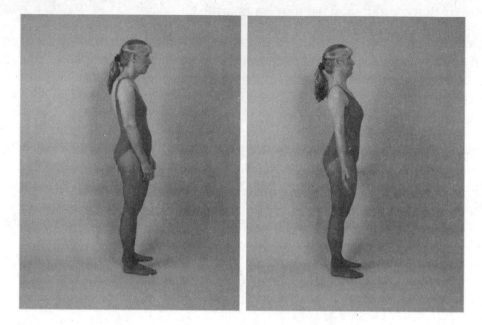

Skeletal Asymmetries

A skeletal asymmetry, including a shorter upper arm and a smaller *hemipelvis* on one side (the left or right portion of the pelvis), can contribute to trigger points in the elbow, lower arm, wrist, or hand. Fortunately these can be corrected inexpensively and noninvasively with a pad that goes on one armrest or other ergonomically correct furniture, or a pad that goes on your chair under one buttock.

Injuries

Injuries are one of the most common initiators of trigger points in general, and one of the more common factors in shoulder, upper arm, or hand muscles specifically. A healthy muscle is pliable to the touch when not in use but will feel firm if called upon for action. If a muscle feels firm at rest, it is tight in an unhealthy way, even if you work out.

I like to use an analogy of a rubber band and a stick. If a sudden, unexpected force is applied to a stick, it's likely to be damaged, and the same is true of a tight muscle, where the force could be something like a fall or a car accident. If, however, a sudden force is applied to a rubber band, it will stretch to absorb the force instead, and the same is true of a pliable, healthy muscle, making it much less likely to be injured. A muscle may be tight and restricted without you being aware of it, since latent trigger points restrict range of motion to some degree and almost everyone has some latent trigger points. Muscles containing latent trigger points can be injured easily if a sudden force is applied.

New Injuries

Treating an injury when it first occurs can prevent trigger points from forming and help you to avoid an escalating cycle of pain. See an acupuncturist or massage therapist who is experienced in working with recent injuries. You may also need to see a chiropractor or osteopathic physician.

Surgeries and Scars

A surgery is likely to leave some scar tissue, which can perpetuate trigger points. Scar tissue can be broken up, to an extent, with vigorous cross-friction massage, a technique in which you rub both of your thumbs in opposing directions back and forth across the scar. However, most people won't work on their own scars vigorously enough due to the pain it causes. You will probably need to see a practitioner for help. Acupuncture can treat scar tissue and help eliminate the pain from trigger points around the area. I recommend using both cross-friction massage and acupuncture rather than just one or the other.

Self-Help Techniques for Acute Injuries and Postsurgery Recovery

RICE:

- **Rest** the affected body part.

- **Ice** can reduce swelling, help prevent bruising, and increase blood flow to the area. You can use a cold compress (cold water with ice cubes in a gallon baggie works well). Or, if it is your lower arm, wrist, or hand, you can submerge it in ice water for as long as you can tolerate the cold; you can pull your arm or hand out of the water and put it back in as needed. Ice off and on for at least forty-eight hours.

- **Compress** the affected area, such as with an ACE bandage (but not so tight as to cut off circulation!). This technique is for acute injuries only, unless otherwise instructed by your medical provider.

- **Elevate** the affected area to reduce bleeding and swelling.

Also:

- Gentle massage strokes on the skin, stroking toward your heart, will improve circulation.

- Cross-friction massage and acupuncture are helpful in healing and reducing scar tissue after swelling and bruising have disappeared.

Buy:

- Get some arnica or Traumeel ointment and oral homeopathics from your local health food stores.

- There are Chinese herbs for traumatic injury, which you can get from your local acupuncture practitioner. Naturopathic doctors will also have herbs and trauma kits. Have these handy in your medicine cabinet in case of unexpected acute injuries, and also if you are planning to have a surgery. They work best when use is started immediately after the injury, and as soon after surgery as possible.

Skeletal Misalignments and Spinal Problems

If vertebrae in your back are chronically out of alignment, the stress placed on muscles due to tightness and pain can cause trigger points to form, which will affect your arms all the way down to your fingers. Be aware that you may also suffer from misalignments in your shoulder, elbow, wrist, and even finger joints. These are usually caused by tight muscles to begin with, so a combined approach of skeletal adjustments plus massage or acupuncture is probably necessary for lasting relief.

Skeletal adjustments can be performed by a chiropractor or osteopathic physician, but be sure you choose one who adjusts bones in extremities, since some do only spinal adjustments. They will likely take X-rays at the initial visit to evaluate your spine and possibly other areas. If you have already had X-rays taken, bring them with you so you can avoid the additional cost and exposure to radiation involved in duplicating X-rays.

Chronic pain from herniated and bulging disks may also lead to formation of trigger points in your entire body. Herniated and bulging disks can be very successfully treated with acupuncture (especially plum blossom technique), but if you don't get some relief fairly quickly, you may want to consider surgery. Spinal surgery has gotten so sophisticated that many surgeries are fairly minor procedures that have you back on your feet the next day. If you have stenosis (a narrowing of the central spinal cord canal or the holes where the nerves come out), acupuncture will help with pain but not the stenosis, so surgery may be the best option. With any surgery, there is a certain amount of risk, so be sure to discuss this with your surgeon and make sure you understand the procedure. If you are still unsure, get a second opinion from another surgeon. Disk problems and stenosis must be confirmed with an MRI. If you have surgery but your pain continues, trigger points are likely to be the culprit, in which case they need to be treated so you can experience lasting relief. If you still don't get relief, the pain may be due to scar tissue from the surgery compressing a nerve root, something you'll need to confirm with your doctor.

Bone spurs and narrowed disk spaces can also cause chronic pain and lead to the formation of trigger points. But in a random sample of the population, you will find many people with bone spurs and narrowed disk spaces who don't experience pain, and many people who do experience pain but don't have bone spurs or narrowed disk spaces. Don't assume these are causing your problems, even if a practitioner has made this assumption.

I always start with the premise that trigger points are at least part of the problem, if not all of the problem, and treat accordingly. If a patient doesn't get some relief fairly quickly, then I know something else may be going on. At that point, I refer them to someone who can evaluate them with an X-ray or MRI.

Conclusion

To address perpetuating factors related to body mechanics, start with changing your workstation. Notice how you are using your body, particularly during work, hobbies, and sports, and be sure not to overdo new exercises. Stretch well before and after athletic activities. Notice how you hold your body, and start retraining yourself to both relax and learn proper posture. Something that may initially seem irrelevant to your situation may lead to a dramatic reduction in the intensity and frequency of your pain. If the self-help techniques aren't effective, consult with a health care professional who can help you to figure out which self-help approaches are most important for you or to get fitted for custom corrective devices.

The next chapter will discuss nutrition and other dietary perpetuating factors.

Chapter 6

Diet

What you eat and drink has a great deal to do with the perpetuation of trigger points. Improving your nutrition, drinking enough water, and avoiding certain foods, drinks, and other substances can greatly decrease trigger point aggravation, and therefore also decrease both the intensity and frequency of your elbow, lower arm, wrist, or hand pain.

Nutritional Deficiencies

It is easy and relatively inexpensive to improve your nutrient intake to see if it will decrease your symptoms. Doctors Travell and Simons (1983) found that almost half of their patients required treatment for vitamin deficiencies to obtain lasting relief from the pain and dysfunction of trigger points. They believed it was one of the most important perpetuating factors to address. The more deficient in nutrients you are, the more symptoms of all kinds.

A *nutrient insufficiency* means that levels are within the lower 25 percent of the normal range, which may cause subtle clinical signs and symptoms. Most health care providers will dismiss lower levels of a vitamin or mineral as being irrelevant, since results are within a "normal" range. However, insufficiencies can cause and perpetuate chronic pain. Several factors may lead to nutrient insufficiency, including inadequate intake of a nutrient, impaired nutrient absorption, inadequate nutrient utilization, increased need by the body, nutrients leaving the body too quickly, and nutrients being destroyed within the body too quickly.

What to Take

Even if you have a fairly healthy diet, you may need supplements. In many places, agricultural soils have been depleted of nutrients by repeatedly planting the same crops in the same location rather than rotating them to replenish the soil. Use of chemical fertilizers and pesticides can also adversely affect both crops and soil, so food doesn't always provide all of the nutrition we require. Shipping food over long distances or storing it for long periods also depletes the nutritive value—too much time passes between when the crop is picked and when it is consumed. Most people need to take some kind of multivitamin and multimineral supplement to ensure proper nutrition, especially those who fall into one of the high-risk groups mentioned later in this chapter.

Don't megadose on supplements unless a doctor has determined your condition warrants it, since taking too much of certain vitamins, such as A, D, E, and folic acid, can actually be detrimental and could cause symptoms similar to deficiencies. You may want to work with a practitioner to develop a personalized supplement program. Some health care providers can arrange for testing to determine any inadequacies. This is especially important because some people aren't able to absorb certain nutrients and need to take them in megadoses or have them injected. For example, some people can't absorb vitamin B_{12}, so they need to get intramuscular injections to ensure adequate levels.

The sections below will discuss the nutrients most likely to be involved in the perpetuation of trigger points. If you have other nutritional concerns or would like more information about any of the nutrients discussed here, *Prescription for Nutritional Healing* by James F. Balch, MD, and Phyllis A. Balch, CNC (2000) is an excellent source. It offers information on vitamins, minerals, amino acids, antioxidants, and enzymes, and it lists food sources for each. Sections on common disorders list supplements useful for treating each condition.

Self-help technique: Take supplements. Because some vitamins require the presence of other vitamins for optimal absorption or effectiveness, taking a good multivitamin supplement and a good multimineral supplement helps ensure that the needed combinations are present. If you take a multivitamin that also includes minerals, check the label to make sure there are adequate amounts of minerals in it; if not, you may need to take a multimineral too. In addition, you might need to take supplements of some of the vitamins and minerals listed below. Doctors Travell and Simons (1983) found that the most important supplements for treating trigger points were the water-soluble vitamins C, B_1, B_6, B_{12}, and folic acid, and the minerals calcium, magnesium, iron, and potassium. The importance of vitamin D has been discovered more recently.

When to Take Supplements

Take your vitamins with food, since some nutrients need to bind with substances found in food in order to be absorbed. You may find that it is best to take your vitamins and herbs when you are not sick, with the exception of herbs specifically made for fighting illness. (See "Acute or

Chronic Infections" in chapter 7 for suggestions on how to head off illness.) Once all of your symptoms have abated, you can resume your regular program of supplementation.

Impaired Digestive Function and Nutrient Malabsorption

If your digestive system isn't functioning well, symptoms may include any of the following: gas, belching, bloating, acid regurgitation, heartburn, diarrhea, constipation, pencil-thin stools, undigested food in your stools, and weight gain even though you're not eating excessively. Taking digestive enzymes or hydrochloric acid for long periods isn't a good solution for poor digestion, because they can take over some of the natural digestive functions of your body. Instead, you need to repair your body so it can do its job properly. A naturopath, acupuncturist, or herbalist can help you figure out whether you have digestive problems. These professionals can also give you dietary recommendations based on your constitution as well as any health problems you might have, and can prescribe herbs to rebalance your system.

Although fasting is often recommended as a way to give the digestive system a rest, it's actually hard on the digestive system. If you want to do a cleanse, use herbs and psyllium, but don't stop eating. Another common misconception is that raw foods and whole grains are the healthiest things to eat. For most foods, it's actually better to cook (not overcook!) them to start the chemical breakdown process so your digestive system doesn't have to work as hard. If you have digestive difficulties, white rice and white bread are easier to digest than whole grain products. As your digestive function heals, your practitioner can recommend the appropriate foods for your constitution.

If you have chronic diarrhea, food won't remain in your intestines long enough for nutrients to be adequately absorbed. You will need to identify and eliminate the source of diarrhea. Acupuncture, herbs, and dietary changes can often successfully address this problem.

I've seen many people who have injured their digestive system by taking too many herbs, or herbs that are inappropriate for their health conditions and constitution. Most herbs should be taken only with the advice of a qualified practitioner. An herb that's beneficial for a friend or a family member may not be appropriate for you.

High-Risk Groups

You may be at a higher risk for nutrient deficiency if you are elderly, pregnant or nursing, poor, depressed, or seriously ill, or if you abuse alcohol or other drugs. If you tend to diet by leaving out important food groups or have an eating disorder, you are also likely to have nutrient deficiencies. And in general, many of us have diets that are neither balanced nor high in nutrition. If you eat a lot of processed foods, be aware that they don't contain as much nutrition as foods that are freshly prepared.

Vegetarianism and Nutrition

Most people should not be strict vegetarians. The forms of B_6 found in animal sources are more stable and less likely to be damaged or lost during cooking or preserving than the main form found in plants. In addition, vitamin B_{12} is found only in animal proteins, including dairy products. Even brewer's yeast doesn't contain B_{12} unless the yeast is grown on a special substrate that contains it.

Self-help technique: Improve your protein intake. If you're vegetarian, at the very least you should eat organic eggs, as they are a source of high-quality protein. Most vegetarians are not very good about combining foods to optimize the balance of *amino acids* (the constituents of protein) in their diet. Even if they are, many report feeling better within a few months when they add high-quality animal protein back into their diet, even if it is just a few eggs or a piece of fish once per week or a couple of times per month.

Vitamins

Adequate intake of vitamin C and D, and the B vitamins is important for resolving trigger points. The B-complex vitamins should be taken together, since they rely on each other for proper absorption and use by your body.

Vitamin C

Vitamin C reduces postexercise soreness and strengthens the capillaries; when these tiny blood vessels are fragile, you'll bruise easily. (Hint: If you don't remember how you got a bruise, you're probably bruising too easily.) Vitamin C is essential for the formation of *collagen* (connective tissue) and bones, and is required for synthesis of the neurotransmitters norepinephrine and serotonin. It is needed for your body's response to stress, plays an important role in immune system function, and decreases the irritability of trigger points caused by infection. Vitamin C helps with diarrhea due to food allergies, but taking too much can lead to watery diarrhea or nonspecific urethritis.

Initial symptoms of vitamin C deficiency include weakness, lethargy, irritability, vague aching pains in the joints and muscles, easy bruising, and possibly weight loss. With severe deficiency (scurvy), the gums become red and swollen and bleed easily, and the teeth may become loose or fall out; however, this condition is rare in most countries with ample access to fruits and vegetables. Vitamin C is likely to be deficient in smokers, alcoholics, older people (the presence of vitamin C in the tissues decreases with age), infants fed primarily on cows' milk (usually between the ages of six and twelve months), people with chronic diarrhea, psychiatric patients, and fad dieters.

Self-help technique: Get enough vitamin C. Good food sources include citrus fruits and fresh juices, raw broccoli, raw Brussels sprouts, collard greens, kale, turnip greens, guava, raw sweet peppers, cabbage, and potatoes. It is currently known that vitamin C daily doses above 400 milligrams (mg) are not used by the body, and that taking 1,000 mg daily increases the risk of kidney stones in people with kidney problems, so megadosing with vitamin C is not necessary (Simons, Travell, and Simons 1999, 207). Women taking estrogen or oral contraceptives may need 500 mg per day. Do not take vitamin C together with antacids. Since vitamin C is ascorbic acid and the purpose of an antacid is to neutralize acid, antacids will neutralize vitamin C and make it ineffective.

Vitamin B$_1$

Vitamin B$_1$ (thiamin) is essential for normal nerve function and the production of energy within muscle cells. Diminished sensitivity to pain and temperature and an inability to detect vibrations are indicators of vitamin B$_1$ deficiency. You may also experience cramping of your calves at night, slight swelling, constipation, and fatigue. B$_1$ is needed for the body to produce adequate amounts of thyroid hormones (for more on this topic, see "Organ Dysfunction and Disease" in chapter 7). Abuse of alcohol reduces absorption of vitamin B$_1$, and liver disease will further reduce absorption. Antacids, the tannins in black tea, or a magnesium deficiency can also prevent the absorption. Because vitamin B$_1$ is water soluble, it will be excreted too rapidly if you're taking diuretics or drinking an excessive amount of water. Vitamin B$_1$ can be destroyed by processing foods, and by heating them to temperatures above 212°F (100°C).

Self-help technique: Get enough vitamin B$_1$. Good food sources include lean pork, kidney, liver, beef, eggs, fish, beans, nuts, and some whole grain cereals, if the hull and germ are present.

Vitamin B$_6$

Vitamin B$_6$ (pyridoxine) is important for nerve function, energy metabolism, amino acid metabolism, and synthesis of neurotransmitters, including norepinephrine and serotonin, which strongly influence pain perception. Deficiency of B$_6$ results in anemia, reduced absorption and storage of B$_{12}$, increased excretion of vitamin C, and blocked synthesis of niacin. It can also lead to a hormonal imbalance. Deficiency of B$_6$ will manifest as symptoms of deficiency of one of the other B vitamins, since B$_6$ is needed for all of the others to perform their functions. The need for B$_6$ increases with age and with eating a high proportion of protein. Tropical spruc (a malabsorption disease) and alcohol use interfere with the body's uptake of B$_6$. Use of oral contraceptives increases your requirement for B$_6$ and leads to impaired glucose tolerance (a prediabetic condition). This can lead to depression if you don't supplement with B$_6$, particularly if you already have a history of depression. Corticosteroid use, excessive alcohol consumption, pregnancy and lactation, antituberculosis drugs, uremia, and hyperthyroidism also increase the need for B$_6$.

Self-help technique: Get enough vitamin B$_6$. Good food sources include liver, kidney, chicken (white meat), halibut, tuna, English walnuts, soybean flour, navy beans, bananas, and avocados, but remember that the forms of B$_6$ found in animal sources are less susceptible to loss due to cooking or preserving than the main form found in plants. There is also some B$_6$ present in yeast, lean beef, egg yolks, and whole wheat.

Vitamin B$_{12}$

Vitamin B$_{12}$ (cyanocobalamin) must be taken together with folic acid in order for the body to form red blood cells and rapidly dividing cells such as those found in the gastrointestinal tract, and for the synthesis of fatty acids used in the formation of parts of certain nerve fibers. B$_{12}$ is also needed for metabolism of both fats and carbohydrates. A deficiency can result in pernicious anemia, a condition that reduces the amount of oxygen available to all of your tissues, including muscles and their trigger points, adding to the cycle of dysfunction and increasing pain. A deficiency of B$_{12}$ may also cause nonspecific depression (depression that isn't temporary and isn't due to a specific event), fatigue, an exaggerated startle reaction to noise or touch, and an increased susceptibility to trigger points. Several drugs may impair the absorption of B$_{12}$, as can megadoses of vitamin C taken for long periods.

Self-help technique: Get enough vitamin B$_{12}$. Animal products and brewer's yeast grown on a special substrate are the only food sources of vitamin B$_{12}$. Strict vegetarians must supplement with this vitamin.

Folate

Folate, also known as folic acid when in the synthetic form, is another member of the B complex. A folate deficiency can cause you to be fatigued easily, sleep poorly, or feel discouraged and depressed. It can also cause restless legs syndrome, diffuse muscular pain, diarrhea, or a loss of sensation in your extremities. You may feel cold frequently and have a slightly lower basal body temperature than the normal 98.6°F (37°C). It can also lead to megaloblastic anemia, a condition where the red blood cells are larger than normal, most often due to a deficiency of folate and/or vitamin B$_{12}$.

In the United States, studies have shown that at least 15 percent of Caucasians are deficient in folate, while at least 30 percent of African-Americans and Latinos are deficient. Part of the problem is that 50 to 95 percent of the folate content of foods may be destroyed during processing and preparation, so even if your diet is rich in foods that are sources of folate, you may not be receiving the benefit (Simons, Travell, and Simons 1999).

Folate is converted into its active form in the digestive system, but this conversion is inhibited by peas, beans, and acidic foods, so eat these separately from your folic acid sources. Those at greatest risk for folate deficiency are the elderly and those who have a bowel disorder, are pregnant or lactating, or use drugs and alcohol regularly. Certain medications deplete folic acid, such as anti-inflammatories (including aspirin), diuretics, estrogens (as in birth control pills and estrogen-based hormone replacement therapy), and anticonvulsants.

Self-help technique: Get enough folate. The best food sources are green leafy vegetables, brewer's yeast, organ meat, fruit, and lightly cooked vegetables such as broccoli and asparagus. As with ascorbic acid (vitamin C), don't take folic acid supplements together with antacids. Also, you must have adequate levels of B_{12} in order to absorb folic acid, and supplementing with only one of these can mask a severe deficiency in the other.

Vitamin D

Vitamin D is required for both the absorption and the utilization of calcium and phosphorus. It is necessary for growth and thyroid function, it protects against muscle weakness, and it helps regulate the heartbeat. It is important for the prevention of cancer, osteoarthritis, osteoporosis, and calcium deficiency. A mild deficiency of vitamin D may manifest as a loss of appetite, a burning sensation in the mouth and throat, diarrhea, insomnia, visual problems, and weight loss. It has been estimated that close to 90 percent of patients with chronic musculoskeletal pain may have a vitamin D deficiency (Heath and Elovic 2006).

Self-Help Technique: Sources of vitamin D include salmon, halibut, sardines, tuna, and eggs. Other sources include dairy products, dandelion greens, liver, oatmeal, and sweet potatoes. If you take supplements, look for the D_3 form, or fish oil capsules.

Vitamin D_3 is synthesized by the skin when exposed to the sun's UV rays. Unfortunately, many people don't get enough sun exposure, especially if they live at latitudes or in climates with little sun available during the winter months. Exposing your face and arms to the sun for fifteen minutes three times per week will ensure that your body synthesizes an adequate amount of vitamin D. Because the amount of exposure needed varies from person to person, and also depends on geographical location, you will need to do some personal research and perhaps consult with a dermatologist to determine the proper amount for you.

Minerals

Calcium, magnesium, potassium, and iron are needed for proper muscle function. Iron is required for transporting oxygen to the muscle fibers. Calcium is essential for releasing acetylcholine at the nerve terminals, and both calcium and magnesium are needed in order for muscle fibers to contract. Potassium is needed to quickly get muscle fibers ready for their next contraction, and a deficiency may cause muscle soreness during exercise or other physical activity. Deficiency of any of these minerals increases the irritability of trigger points. Calcium, magnesium, and potassium should be taken together, because an increase in one by itself can deplete the others.

Salt is another important mineral. Don't entirely eliminate it from your diet, especially if you sweat. You do need some salt in your diet, unless you have been instructed otherwise by your doctor for certain medical conditions. Inadequate levels of sodium, calcium, magnesium, or potassium can lead to muscle cramping.

Calcium

Tums or other antacids can't substitute for calcium supplements, because they neutralize stomach acid, which is needed for the uptake of calcium. If you must take an antacid, take your calcium-magnesium supplement several hours before or afterward to maximize your absorption. Vitamin D_3 is needed for calcium uptake. It is especially important to take calcium for at least a few years prior to menopause to help prevent osteoporosis.

Calcium channel blockers prescribed for high blood pressure inhibit the uptake of calcium into the sarcoplasmic reticulum of vascular smooth muscles and cardiac muscles. Since this is probably also true for skeletal muscles, calcium channel blockers are likely to aggravate trigger points and make them more difficult to treat. If you're taking calcium channel blockers, ask your doctor whether you can switch to a different medication. Consider treating the underlying causes of your high blood pressure with acupuncture, dietary changes, exercise, or whatever is appropriate to your particular set of circumstances.

Self-help technique: Get enough calcium. Good food sources include salmon, sardines, other seafood, green leafy vegetables, almonds, asparagus, blackstrap molasses, brewer's yeast, broccoli, cabbage, carob, collard greens, dandelion greens, figs, filberts, kale, kelp, mustard greens, oats, parsley, prunes, sesame seeds, tofu, and turnip greens. Dairy products and whey are also good sources, but they're contraindicated if you have fibromyalgia or a "damp-type condition" as diagnosed by traditional Chinese medicine.

Magnesium

If you have a healthy diet, you're probably getting enough magnesium; any deficiency is probably due to malabsorption, kidney disease, or fluid and electrolyte loss. Magnesium is depleted after strenuous physical exercise, but reasonable amounts of exercise coupled with an adequate intake of magnesium will improve the efficiency of cellular metabolism and improve your cardiorespiratory performance. Consumption of alcohol, use of diuretics, chronic diarrhea, or consumption of fluoride or high amounts of zinc and vitamin D increase the body's need for magnesium.

Self-help technique: Get enough magnesium. Magnesium is found in most foods, especially meat, fish and other seafood, apples, apricots, avocados, bananas, blackstrap molasses, brewer's yeast, brown rice, figs, garlic, kelp, lima beans, millet, nuts, peaches, black-eyed peas, sesame seeds, tofu, green leafy vegetables, wheat, and whole grains. Dairy products are also good sources, but they're contraindicated if you have fibromyalgia or a "damp-type condition" as diagnosed by traditional Chinese medicine. If you are an athlete, you will probably want to take additional magnesium supplements.

Potassium

A diet high in fats, refined sugars, and salt causes potassium deficiency, as does the use of laxatives and some diuretics. Diarrhea will also deplete potassium. If you experience urinary frequency, particularly if your urine is clear rather than light yellow, try taking potassium. Frequent urination causes potassium deficiency, and because potassium deficiency may, in turn, cause frequent urination, a self-perpetuating cycle can ensue.

Self-help technique: Get enough potassium. Good food sources include fruit (especially bananas and citrus fruits), potatoes, green leafy vegetables, wheat germ, beans, lentils, nuts, dates, and prunes.

Iron

Iron deficiency, which can lead to anemia, is usually caused by excessive blood loss from heavy menses, hemorrhoids, intestinal bleeding, donating blood too often, or ulcers. Iron deficiency can also be caused by a long-term illness, prolonged use of antacids, poor digestion, excessive consumption of coffee or black tea, or the chronic use of NSAIDs (nonsteroidal anti-inflammatory drugs, such as ibuprofen). Early symptoms of iron deficiency include fatigue, reduced endurance, and an inability to stay warm when exposed to a moderately cold environment. Between 9 and 11 percent of menstruating females in the United States are iron deficient, and the worldwide prevalence is about 15 percent (Simons, Travell, and Simons 1999).

If you believe you suffer from an iron deficiency, see your doctor. You shouldn't take iron supplements unless prescribed, other than what is found in a multivitamin or multimineral, because there are health risks associated with taking too much iron. Also, don't take an iron supplement if you have an infection or cancer. The body stores it in order to withhold it from bacteria, and in the case of cancer, it may suppress the cancer-killing function of certain cells.

Self-help technique: Get enough iron—but not too much. Iron is best absorbed with vitamin C. For most people, food sources are adequate for improving iron levels. Good sources include eggs, fish, liver, meat, poultry, green leafy vegetables, whole grains, almonds, avocados, beets, blackstrap molasses, brewer's yeast, dates, egg yolks, kelp, kidney and lima beans, lentils, millet, parsley, peaches, pears, prunes, pumpkin, raisins, sesame seeds, and soybeans. Calcium in milk and other dairy products, or a calcium supplement, can impair absorption of iron, so you should take calcium supplements at a different time than iron supplements.

Water

It's important to drink enough water, because water is the lubricating fluid of your body. Would you drive your car without oil in it? Dehydration is especially common among people who take diuretic medications or drink a lot of coffee or other beverages with diuretic qualities. Don't drink distilled water or rainwater, because you need the minerals found in nondistilled water. If you drink bottled water, know the source of the water to make sure it's not distilled or the minerals otherwise removed. This industry currently isn't regulated, so you may need to do some research on the company.

Self-help technique: Drink enough water. Drink about two quarts of water per day, and more if you have a larger body mass or sweat a lot. Here's a general rule of thumb for people weighing more than 100 pounds: divide your body weight by two, and drink that number of ounces each day. So if you weigh 140 pounds, you should be drinking seventy ounces. Drink at least one extra quart per day if it is very hot out, and drink extra water during and immediately after a workout. Drinking too much water is not advisable, since you can deplete vitamin B_1 (thiamin) and other water-soluble vitamins. Also, room-temperature water is better than cold; if you drink something cold, your stomach has to expend energy to warm it up, so it taxes your digestive system.

Improper Diet

Eating foods that aggravate trigger points is a common and significant perpetuating factor. Depending on your constitution, health conditions, and any food allergies, avoiding certain foods can help enormously in relieving your pain.

Plan on avoiding the foods and substances indicated below for at least two months, in conjunction with receiving acupuncture treatments and/or taking herbs and other supplements, in order to determine whether eliminating the specific item is helpful. Many people will stop consuming a food or other substance for just a short while, perhaps only a week, then decide it hasn't made a difference and start consuming those substances again. Or the foods, beverages, or other substances may be so important to them that they'd rather have pain and other medical conditions than give the substances up. Reaching a conclusion after only a short trial period is one way to justify continuing to consume something that causes you problems.

Foods and Drinks to Avoid

You may be reluctant to give up a favorite food or beverage. However, I suggest you read this section and consider that the listed items could be at least part of the cause of your pain. Then you can make an informed decision about how committed you are to getting rid of your pain.

Caffeine

Caffeine causes a persistent contracture of muscle fibers (sometimes referred to as "caffeine rigor") and increases muscle tension and trigger point irritability, leading to an increase in pain. It causes excessive amounts of calcium to be released from the sarcoplasmic reticulum and interferes with the rebinding of calcium ions by the sarcoplasmic reticulum. Doctors Travell and Simons (1983) found that caffeine in excess of 150 mg daily (more than two eight-ounce cups of regular coffee) would lead to caffeine rigor. I suspect for some people it could be even less. In assessing your daily intake, be sure to count any caffeine in tea, sodas, and other beverages, and in any drugs you may be taking, and remember that espresso and similar drinks have more concentrated amounts of caffeine.

Alcohol, Tobacco, and Marijuana

Alcohol aggravates trigger points by decreasing serum and tissue levels of folate. It increases the body's need for vitamin C while decreasing the body's ability to absorb it. Tobacco also increases the need for vitamin C.

In traditional Chinese medicine, caffeine and alcohol are said to be very "qi stagnating." The ancient concept of qi is not easily translatable into Western medical terminology. It is thought that qi is energy that flows through fourteen main "meridians" and connecting vessels that go to all parts of the body. Qi moves the blood and lymph fluids. When the flow of qi is blocked (stagnation), pain and disease result. Based on today's understanding of body processes, some think that qi refers to the biochemical processes in living creatures—the combination of electrical impulses, neurotransmitters, hormones, body fluids, and cellular metabolism that allow us to be living, breathing creatures. As you read in chapter 1, trigger points form when your fluids aren't moving well, cellular metabolism isn't working properly, and neurotransmitters aren't operating normally, which supports that particular concept of qi, and the idea of pain resulting from qi stagnation.

Marijuana is also very stagnating, and it stays in your system for about three months after smoking it. Stagnation is one cause of pain; therefore, using any of these substances will increase your pain level.

Food Allergies

Exposure to both environmental and food-related allergens causes the body to release histamines, which perpetuates trigger points and makes them harder to treat. Avoiding allergenic foods can be challenging when you're dining out, traveling, or eating at someone else's home. Whenever it's feasible, bring along something you can eat so you'll have an alternative.

Self-help technique: Do a self-test for food allergens. There are a few methods of testing for food allergens. One of the best ways is an elimination diet, where you eliminate all suspect foods, then add them back in one at a time, and then rotate foods. You can find instructions for this in *Prescription for Nutritional Healing* (Balch and Balch 2000), under "Allergies." However, most people aren't willing to take this approach, as it requires you to be very disciplined about your diet and keep a careful food diary for a month. As an alternative, *Prescription for Nutritional Healing* offers a quick test. After sitting and relaxing for a few minutes, take your pulse rate for one minute, and then eat the food you are testing. Keep still for fifteen to twenty minutes and take your pulse again. If your pulse rate has increased more than ten beats per minute, eliminate this food from your diet for one month, then retest. Another option is a blood test for food allergens, offered by naturopaths and some other practitioners.

Conclusion

Improving your nutrition, changing your diet, and avoiding detrimental foods, beverages, and inhaled substances will likely take some time, but you can start by taking a multivitamin and multimineral supplement and drinking enough water. As you identify which foods you need to avoid, start replacing them with foods high in the vitamins and minerals discussed in this chapter. Be sure you are getting enough protein.

The next chapter covers the remaining perpetuating factors that are most likely to cause and perpetuate trigger points, including emotional factors, sleep problems, acute and chronic infections, hormonal imbalances, and organ dysfunction and disease.

Chapter 7

Other Perpetuating Factors

Several other factors that can perpetuate trigger points are worth mentioning, since they may play an important role in your elbow, lower arm, wrist, or hand pain. Emotional factors such as anxiety and depression, sleep problems, acute and chronic infections, hormonal imbalances, and organ dysfunction and disease can all be involved in the formation and perpetuation of trigger points. Laboratory tests are required to diagnose some of these conditions, so you'll probably need to work with a doctor to determine whether those factors are involved in causing your trigger points.

Emotional Factors

Emotional factors can contribute greatly to causing and perpetuating pain—and many other health conditions as well. As you may recall from chapter 1, while prolonged exposure to both emotional and physical stressors can lead to central nervous system sensitization and subsequently cause pain, prolonged pain itself can also lead to central nervous system sensitization, leading to emotional and physical stress (Niddam 2009). Also remember that once the central nervous system is sensitized, pain can be more easily triggered by lower levels of physical and emotional stressors and be more intense and last longer (Latremoliere and Woolf 2009).

While it's encouraging that modern medicine has accepted the role of emotional factors, all too often people are dismissed by their doctors as "just being under stress." The appointment ends and their physical symptoms are neither assessed nor addressed. This is particularly true when it comes to pain and depression. If you're in pain long enough, of course you'll begin to feel fatigued, depressed, and anxious. The converse is also true: if you're depressed, anxious, and fatigued long enough, you'll probably develop pain. It's important to recognize the role of stress and emotional factors as both a cause of illness and a result of illness, and to address them just as you would any other factor.

Depression

If you experience an unusual desire to be alone, a loss of interest in your favorite activities, and a decrease in job performance, and are neglecting your appearance and hygiene, you may be suffering from more than a mild and temporary situation-dependent depression. Clinical symptoms of depression are insomnia, loss of appetite, weight loss, impotence or decreased libido, blurred vision, a sad mood, thoughts of suicide or death, an inability to concentrate, poor memory, indecision, mumbled speech, and negative reactions to suggestions. There can certainly be other reasons for some of these symptoms, and no single symptom is indicative of depression. It is the number and combination of symptoms that leads to a diagnosis of clinical depression. However, if you are having thoughts of suicide or self-harm for any reason, it is imperative that you seek help immediately.

Depression lowers your pain threshold, increases the amount of pain you feel, and adversely affects your response to trigger point therapy. There are many approaches to treating depression (see below), including medications. While antidepressants may help with the acute symptoms, many of them have side effects. Plus, some medications can exacerbate the underlying condition causing the symptoms, so a vicious cycle ensues.

Anxiety

If you are extremely anxious, chances are you're holding tension in at least some of your muscles and developing trigger points as a result. Holding tension in your back, shoulders, and gluteal muscles affects your legs both indirectly through central sensitization and directly through referral patterns that extend into your legs.

Self-help technique: Get help for emotional factors. If you are depressed or anxious, you need to address this in order to speed your recovery from pain. Unfortunately people suffering from severe depression, anxiety, chronic fatigue, or extreme pain often don't have the energy to participate in their own healing. You may have difficulty summoning the energy to cook healthy foods or even get out of bed, and you may not be able to manage to do even mild forms of exercise, such as walking—the very things that would help you start to feel better. You may have a hard time making it to appointments with a counselor or health care practitioner. If this describes you, you need to do whatever you can to get to the point where you can start taking better care of yourself. This may mean taking homeopathic remedies, receiving acupuncture treatments or counseling, or doing the self-help techniques in this book. You may need to take antidepressants or pain relievers for a while until you feel well enough to start using the above suggestions. Just doing one of these things will help get you started in the right direction and improve your energy and outlook.

One of the things I like most about Oriental medicine and homeopathy is that both assume you can't separate the physical body from the emotions. These systems of healing consider both physical and emotional symptoms in developing a diagnosis, and both types of symptoms are treated simultaneously. With acupuncture, there are no side effects and response is usually rapid. With both homeopathy and herbs, the wrong prescription or dosage can have side effects, just as with allopathic prescription drugs, so it is important to consult with a trained professional. Detailed recommendations for treating either depression or anxiety are beyond the scope of this book, but many excellent self-help books on the topic are available. Also see the section on the thyroid in "Organ Dysfunction and Disease" later in this chapter, since thyroid problems can be an undiagnosed cause of depression.

Self-help technique: Get enough exercise. Exercise increases levels of serotonin, a neurotransmitter believed to play an important role in many body functions, including mood regulation. Walking and deep breathing are great for relieving tension, anxiety, and depression. Even walking ten minutes per day can be extremely beneficial, especially if you can walk outside.

Self-help technique: Notice when you're tensing—and relax! Notice whether you're hiking your shoulders up or tightening muscles, particularly when you're under stress. Take a minute to mentally assess your body, noticing where you're holding tension. Whenever you come to an area that's tense, take a deep breath and consciously relax the area as you exhale. Do this several times each day. You will need to retrain yourself to break the habit of holding tension in certain areas.

Sleep Problems

Sleep disorders, interrupted sleep, and insufficient sleep can all perpetuate trigger points, and both the trigger points themselves and the lack of sleep can contribute to pain. The first step in solving this problem is to consider whether you had sleep problems before your elbow, lower arm, wrist, or hand pain started. If you did, then the underlying factors responsible for your sleep problems must be addressed.

Self-help technique: Treat your pain. If pain disturbs you at night, use the self-treatments described in part III to work on your trigger points when you're awakened by pain. Hopefully this will allow you to fall back to sleep once your pain abates. If you're using a ball for self-treatment, as described in part III, don't fall asleep on the ball, since doing so will cut off the circulation for too long and make the trigger points worse.

Self-help technique: Check your environment. Be sure you aren't sleeping poorly due to being too warm or too cold. Fortunately this is relatively easy to address. If noise is waking you, try wearing earplugs. My favorite type is Mack's Pillow Soft silicone earplugs. Computer use or possibly watching TV in the evening can overstimulate the brain and make it hard to fall asleep and sleep restfully.

Make sure you aren't being exposed to allergens at night. Many people are allergic to dust mites, which live in bedding, among other places. An inexpensive solution is to use soft vinyl covers over your pillows and mattress. If you have a down comforter or pillow, you may be allergic to the feathers even if you aren't exhibiting classic allergy symptoms, such as sneezing and itchy eyes. Or it may be that your mattress is worn out, or that your mattress or pillows are inappropriate for your body. See "Misfitting Furniture" in chapter 5 for more information and recommendations.

Self-help technique: Try acupuncture, herbs, or other supplements. Acupuncture and Chinese herbs may be helpful, especially if your mind is overactive, you sleep lightly and wake frequently, you wake up early and can't fall back to sleep, you have vivid and disturbing dreams, or you're menopausal. If urinary frequency is disturbing your sleep, try acupuncture, herbs, and increasing your potassium intake. If you have problems falling asleep, try improving your diet, taking supplements, and drinking enough water—but don't drink too much just before bedtime! Taking a calcium-magnesium supplement before bedtime can be especially helpful, particularly if you are also experiencing muscle cramps.

Self-help technique: Eliminate caffeine and alcohol. Caffeine and alcohol will disturb your sleep or make you sleep more lightly, in addition to aggravating trigger points (see chapter 6). Even if you drink caffeine only in the morning, it can still disrupt your nighttime sleep patterns. If you choose to give up caffeine, you may experience various withdrawal symptoms, and the first few days can be difficult. It will take about two weeks before your energy starts to even out and you feel like you don't need caffeine to get going in the morning.

Self-help technique: Rest and relax more. If you are continually under stress, or if you're pushing yourself too hard and push through fatigue instead of resting or taking a nap, your adrenal glands will excrete excessive amounts of adrenaline, which can interfere with sleep. A naturopathic doctor can administer a saliva test for adrenal function. Try breathing deeply until you fall asleep.

Acute or Chronic Infections

Infections are trigger point perpetuators that are often overlooked, even by experienced health care providers.

Acute Infections

Try to head off acute illnesses, such as colds and flu, at the first sign in order to avoid perpetuating trigger points. This is particularly important if you have fibromyalgia, sinusitis, asthma, or recurrent infections, since your trigger points will be activated by illness. Getting sick can set you back by months in your treatment and healing.

Self-help technique: Don't get sick. With lifestyle modifications and preventive care, it is possible to reduce your incidence of illness. When you start to get sick, take echinacea, the Chinese herbal formulas Gan Mao Ling or Yin Chiao, and/or homeopathic remedies as appropriate, such as Oscillococcinum for flu. Keep these herbs and remedies on hand at home so you can take them as soon as you notice the first signs of illness. Once you're past the initial stage of illness, the herbs or remedies you need will depend on your particular set of symptoms, so you may need to consult with a practitioner.

Chronic Infections

Chronic infections such as sinus infections, urinary tract infections, and herpes simplex (cold sores, genital herpes, or shingles) will perpetuate trigger points, so you need to resolve or manage chronic infections to obtain lasting relief from elbow, lower arm, wrist, and hand pain, and from trigger points in general.

With both sinus infections and urinary tract infections, antibiotics often don't kill all of the pathogens, and you end up with lingering, recurrent infections. However, antibiotics have the advantage of working quickly, so I often recommend combining antibiotics with other treatments, such as acupuncture, herbs, and homeopathic remedies. This will knock the infection out as quickly and completely as possible, and help prevent it from becoming a chronic problem. Urinary tract infections must be dealt with promptly. You can use over-the-counter allopathic drugs, Chinese herbs, or cranberry extract or juice (don't use sweetened juice), but if your symptoms don't improve right away, you need to see your doctor. Urinary tract infections can turn into life-threatening kidney infections very rapidly.

A variety of supplements, herbs, and pharmaceutical drugs are used to treat recurrent herpes infections, and some will work better than others for you. If you have recurrent outbreaks, you need to figure out what is impairing your immune system, such as allergies or emotional stress. Sometimes a herpes outbreak is the first sign that your body is fighting an acute illness. This can be a signal to you to take the remedies mentioned above.

Parasitic Infections

The fish tapeworm, giardia, and the amoeba are the parasites most likely to perpetuate trigger points. The fish tapeworm and giardia both scar the lining of the intestines and impair your ability to absorb nutrients, and they also consume vitamin B_{12}. Amoebas can produce toxins that are passed from the intestines into the rest of the body. Fish tapeworms can be present in raw fish. Giardia is most often associated with drinking untreated water from streams, but it can also be passed by an infected person who doesn't wash their hands after a bowel movement, particularly if they are preparing food or have some other hand-to-mouth contact.

If you have chronic diarrhea, it is worth testing for parasites. However, such tests can be costly, and different tests are required to rule out different parasites. A cheaper alternative is to treat a suspected parasitic infection with herbs like grapefruit seed extract or pulsatilla (a Chinese herb) and see if your symptoms improve. However, if you have blood in your stools, you should see your doctor immediately to rule out serious conditions.

Many people report feeling much better on an anticandida diet, and in any case it is a pretty healthy way to eat. The basics of the diet are to avoid sugar in all its forms, simple and processed carbohydrates, fermented foods, yeast, mushrooms, and certain cheeses. There are many herbal products on the market for eliminating candida, including grapefruit seed extract, oil of oregano, echinacea, pulsatilla, and a variety of formulas. Since most of these will also kill off your beneficial intestinal flora, you need to use a good multiacidophilus supplement after treatment, as you would after taking any antibiotic.

Organ Dysfunction and Disease

Organ dysfunction and disease, such as hypothyroidism, hypometabolism, hypoglycemia, diabetes, and gout, can cause and perpetuate trigger points. Even though these are among the more challenging perpetuating factors to address, treating them is absolutely essential for pain relief.

Thyroid

Both subclinical hypothyroidism (also known as hypometabolism or thyroid inadequacy) and hypothyroidism will cause and perpetuate trigger points. People who have a low-functioning thyroid gland may experience early-morning stiffness and pain and weakness of the shoulder girdle. Symptoms of both subclinical hypothyroidism and hypothyroidism include intolerance to cold (and sometimes heat), cold hands and feet, muscle aches and pains (especially with cold, rainy weather), constipation, menstrual problems, weight gain, dry skin, fatigue, and lethargy. Muscles feel rather hard to the touch, and even if people with hypothyroidism take a thyroid supplement, I've noticed they are still somewhat prone to trigger points, probably because it's hard to fine-tune the dosage to the exact amount the person's body would produce if the thyroid gland were healthy.

Some studies report that as many as 17 percent of women and 7 percent of men have subclinical hypothyroidism (Simons, Travell, and Simons 1999). Contrary to the usual symptoms, some people with subclinical hypothyroidism may be thin, nervous, and hyperactive, and in these cases practitioners may not consider the possibility of hypometabolism.

People with low thyroid function may be low in vitamin B_1 (thiamin). Before starting on thyroid medication, try supplementing with B_1 to see if that corrects your thyroid hormone levels. If you are already on thyroid medication and you start taking B_1, you may develop symptoms of hyperthyroidism, in which case your medication dosage must be adjusted. If you are low in B_1 when you start taking thyroid medication, you may develop symptoms of acute B_1 deficiency, which may be misinterpreted as an intolerance to the medication. After the B_1 deficiency is corrected, you will likely tolerate the medication. You need to supplement with B_1 prior to and during thyroid hormone therapy to avoid a deficiency. Total body potassium is low in hypothyroidism and high in hyperthyroidism, so you may need to adjust your potassium intake as well.

Smoking impairs the action of thyroid hormones and will make any related symptoms worse. Several pharmaceutical drugs, such as lithium, anticonvulsants, glucocorticoid steroids, and drugs that contain iodine, can also affect thyroid hormone levels. If you've been diagnosed with hypothyroidism and are taking other medications, consult with your doctor or pharmacist to see whether any of your medications could be causing the problem.

Self-help technique: Test your thyroid function at home. A simple home test to check your thyroid function is to measure your basal body temperature. Place a thermometer in your armpit for ten minutes upon waking and before getting out of bed. Normal underarm temperature for men and postmenopausal women is 98°F (36.7°C). For premenopausal women, it's 97.5°F (36.4°C) prior to ovulation and 98.5°F (36.9°C) after ovulation. If your temperature is lower than this, consult with your doctor.

Self-help technique: Get the right tests. Often doctors initially test only TSH (thyroid-stimulating hormone) levels. The results may still be normal if you have subclinical hypothyroidism rather than clinical hypothyroidism. A radioimmunoassay measures levels of two specific thyroid hormones—T3 and T4—and gives a more complete picture of your thyroid function. If you are depressed, insist that your thyroid levels be tested before you start taking antidepressant medication. If thyroid dysfunction is responsible for your depression, correcting it may resolve the depression, allowing you to avoid antidepressants and their many side effects. I've had more than one patient (especially men) whose hypothyroidism was discovered only after they had been medicated with antidepressants for some time.

Hypoglycemia

Hypoglycemia is an abnormally low level of glucose in the blood. This is most often related to diabetes, but there are several other, less common possible causes. A hypoglycemic reaction when a meal is delayed (fasting hypoglycemia) usually indicates a problem with the liver, adrenal glands, or pituitary gland. Missing or delaying a meal won't cause hypoglycemia in a healthy person. Onset of hypoglycemia after a meal (reactive hypoglycemia) usually occurs two to three hours after eating a meal rich in carbohydrates and is most likely to occur when you are under a lot of stress. You need to identify the causes and address them if possible.

If you've been diagnosed with hypoglycemia, you probably know the cause and whether it is reactive or fasting hypoglycemia. The important thing to know is that both types cause and perpetuate trigger points and make trigger points more difficult to treat. Symptoms of both types are sweating, trembling and shakiness, increased heart rate, and anxiety. If allowed to progress, symptoms of severe hypoglycemia can include visual disturbances, restlessness, and impaired speech and thinking. Avoid all caffeine, alcohol, and tobacco (even secondhand smoke). Normally the liver converts the body's stored carbohydrates into glucose when blood glucose levels drop, and this helps avoid or slow down a hypoglycemic reaction. However, when you ingest alcohol, caffeine, or tobacco, your liver considers detoxifying your bloodstream the highest priority and will not put more glucose into the bloodstream until it is done, resulting in a hypoglycemic reaction.

Self-help technique: Eat small, frequent meals. Symptoms of hypoglycemia will be relieved by eating smaller, more frequent meals with fewer carbohydrates, more protein, and some fat. If you are waking up with pain or are having trouble sleeping, eating a small snack or drinking a little juice before you go to bed may help. Also, acupuncture is quite successful in stabilizing blood sugar.

Gout

Gout is a disease characterized by high uric acid levels in the blood. It is caused by dietary factors, genetics, or the underexcretion of urate (the salts of uric acid). Monosodium urate (MSU) crystals form and are deposited in joints, tendons, and the surrounding tissues, which usually causes swelling and intense pain due to an inflammatory reaction. The joint at the base of the big toe is most commonly affected, but symptoms can manifest in the wrists or hands too. Gout often occurs in combination with obesity, diabetes, hypertension, insulin resistance, and/or abnormal lipid levels.

Gout will aggravate trigger points and make them difficult to treat. While Doctors Travell and Simons did not speculate in their books as to why gout is a perpetuating factor for trigger points, it is likely that trigger points are caused and perpetuated by the high acid content, in addition to causing a self-perpetuating cycle of pain from central sensitization. (See "Elevated Biochemicals" in chapter 1). Though you may experience only the most obvious symptoms in one of the joints in the lower or upper extremities, because it is a systemic disease, it no doubt affects all muscle tissues.

Conclusion

Eliminating perpetuating factors may possibly give you complete relief from pain without any additional treatment. If you don't resolve or avoid perpetuating factors to the extent possible, you may not get more than temporary relief from any form of treatment.

Hopefully you've learned enough about your potential perpetuating factors that even if you choose not to resolve them, you'll be making an informed choice about which you value more: relief from your elbow, lower arm, wrist, or hand pain, or continuing to do things that make you feel worse, even if they are within your power to change. You will have more control over some perpetuating factors than others. For example, you may not be able to control whether you have hypothyroidism, but you can take thyroid hormones and supplements and stop smoking. Much or all of your elbow, lower arm, wrist, or hand pain is probably within your control. What are you willing to do to change your life?

The next section will teach you how to work on your own trigger points, how to stretch properly, how to care for your muscles, and what you should avoid doing so that you don't make yourself feel worse.

Part III

TRIGGER POINT SELF-HELP TECHNIQUES

In this section, you'll learn how to relieve your trigger points with self-help techniques. Chapter 8 provides general guidelines on how to do trigger point self-treatments and what to avoid, as well as some do's and don'ts for stretching and conditioning. Chapter 9 helps you determine which trigger points cause your elbow, lower arm, wrist, or hand pain. Each of the remaining chapters covers a muscle or group of muscles that may contain trigger points which can contribute to elbow, lower arm, wrist, or hand pain.

In the muscle chapters, anatomical drawings are provided to help you locate where trigger points are most likely located in the muscle and to see what the muscle looks like. Symptom lists and photographs showing pain referral patterns, and lists of common causes and perpetuating factors for trigger points, will help you determine whether a given trigger point might be causing your pain. These are followed by helpful hints for dealing with those causes. Photographs and written instructions provide guidance on self-treatment of trigger points. Most of the muscle chapters also include stretches. Each muscle chapter will also advise you to check other muscles that may be involved.

Chapter 8

General Guidelines
for Self-Treatment

In this chapter, you'll learn how to apply pressure to trigger points and how to stretch and condition muscles properly. I'll also offer general guidelines on caring for your muscles in order to prevent the reactivation of trigger points.

General Guidelines for Applying Pressure During Self-Treatments

Applying pressure on your own trigger points can give you a great deal of relief within the first few weeks, but you must perform the techniques properly. You can expect gradual improvement over a period of days and weeks. Review the following guidelines frequently in the beginning stages of treatment, and then periodically to ensure you are performing the techniques properly.

How Not to Perform Self-Treatments

The most important guideline is this: don't overdo it! Many people think that if some self-treatment feels good, doing it harder, longer, or more often will be even more helpful. But you can actually make yourself worse by doing treatments too frequently or doing them incorrectly.

Don't apply pressure over varicose veins, open wounds, infected areas, herniated or bulging disks, areas affected by phlebitis or thrombophlebitis, or anywhere clots are present or could be present. If you're pregnant, don't apply pressure on your legs.

If your symptoms get worse or you are sore from treatments for more than one day, stop the self-treatments for a few days until your symptoms improve, then resume doing the treatments less frequently and using less pressure to see if you can tolerate them without feeling worse or sore. Chances are you were using too much pressure or holding the points for too long. Review these guidelines if that is the case. If you're seeing a practitioner, they may be able to help you figure out any problems with how you are doing the self-treatments. And if you are sore from a therapist's work, be sure to tell them.

How to Work on Trigger Points

The most important technique for treating trigger points, other than eliminating perpetuating factors, is applying pressure. Use a tennis ball, racquetball, golf ball, dog play ball, or baseball, or use your elbow or hand if instructed to do so for particular muscles. When lying on balls, use only the weight of your body to give you pressure. Don't actively press your back or other body parts onto the balls. The muscle you're working on should be as passive as possible. Use only one ball at a time on your back, not one on each side. If you need to work on your back muscles during the workday, I recommend getting a Backnobber, a large S-shaped gadget for applying pressure, available from the Pressure Positive Company (see Resources) and other sources.

Apply pressure for a minimum of eight seconds (less than that may activate trigger points) and a maximum of one minute (to avoid cutting off the circulation for too long, which could aggravate the trigger point). You can count out the time by saying "one one thousand, two one thousand, three one thousand," and so on. Time yourself first to be sure you are actually counting seconds at the correct speed; don't race to eight as quickly as possible.

The pressure should be somewhat uncomfortable but hurt in a good way. It shouldn't be so painful that you tense up or hold your breath. If you're using a ball and the treatment is too painful, move to a softer surface such as a bed, or pad the surface with a pillow or blanket. Alternatively, try using a smaller or softer ball. You can puncture a tennis ball with a nail to make it softer. If the treatment doesn't produce tenderness at all, keep looking for tender spots or try moving to a harder surface. If you're using a ball for treatment but the trigger point is too tender for you to lie on it at all, try putting the ball in a long sock and leaning against the wall. However, I recommend this only if you can't lie on the ball, since leaning against the wall involves using the very muscles you are trying to work on. You may need to use a combination of surfaces depending on the tenderness of different areas. Over time, as your sensitivity decreases and you're able to work the deeper parts of the muscle, you may need to use a ball that's harder or a different size, or to move to a harder surface. Experiment to find what's effective for you.

If your time is limited, treat one area thoroughly rather than rushing through many areas. If you hurry, you're more likely to aggravate trigger points rather than inactivate them.

If you're using a ball for self-treatment, be careful not to fall asleep on the ball, since doing so will cut off the circulation for too long and make the trigger points worse. When you're fatigued and in pain and suddenly the pain is reduced or gone, it's all too easy to fall asleep on the ball, so don't use this technique in bed unless you're sure that won't happen.

Where to Find Trigger Points

Search the entire muscle, particularly the points of maximum tenderness, to make sure you find all the potential trigger points. Use the muscle drawings and pictures in the following chapters to make sure you're searching the entire muscle and not just focusing on the most painful spot. Many times a tendon attachment will hurt because the tight muscle is pulling on it, but if you don't work on the entire belly of the muscle, it will keep pulling on the attachment.

If you find trigger points on one side of the body, be sure to work on the same muscles on the other side, but spend more time on the side that's causing your pain. Except for very new one-sided injuries, the same muscle on the opposite side will almost always also be tender with applied pressure, even if it hasn't started causing symptoms yet. For back muscles, loosening one side but not the other can lead to new problems. And sometimes the muscles on the opposite side are actually causing the symptoms, so it's always worthwhile to work on both sides.

Pressure on a trigger point may reproduce the referred pain pattern, but this doesn't always occur. So if you have reason to suspect that a particular muscle is involved, work on it anyway and see if it helps relieve your pain and other symptoms. If you improve, even temporarily, assume that one of the trigger points you worked on is indeed at least part of the problem. For this reason, don't work on all the possible trigger points in one session, since you won't know which trigger point treated actually gave you relief.

Work in the direction of referral. For example, if trigger points in the infraspinatus muscle are referring pain to your arm and hand, work first on the infraspinatus muscle (over the back of shoulder blade), then the upper arm, then the lower arm, and then the hand.

If treatments seem effective but you get only temporary relief, start searching for trigger points that refer pain or other symptoms to the area you've already located and treated for trigger points. It may be that you have been working on satellite trigger points and need to locate the primary trigger points that are activating the satellite trigger points. You can't resolve satellite trigger points without first addressing the primary trigger points causing them. For example, if you have pain down the back of your upper and lower arm, and possibly into the hand, and you can get only temporary relief by working on the coracobrachialis muscle, consider whether referral from primary trigger points in the deltoid, pectoralis major, latissimus dorsi, teres major, supraspinatus, triceps, and/or biceps muscles are keeping the satellite coracobrachialis trigger points active.

Each muscle chapter contains a list of other muscles that may also be involved (under "Also See"). However, because each person's body is so different, you may need to look through the referral patterns in all of the muscle chapters to determine which other muscles may be involved in your case.

Frequency of Self-Treatments

Most people should work on their muscles one time per day initially. Pick a time when you'll remember to do your self-treatments—perhaps when you wake up, when you watch television, or when you go to bed—and keep your balls where they'll be handy. (Just be careful not to fall asleep on a ball!) If you're sore from self-treatments or your practitioner's treatments, skip a day. If you're seeing a practitioner, don't do self-treatments on the same day you have an appointment.

After a few weeks, you can increase your self-treatments to twice per day as long as you're not getting sore. If a particular activity seems to aggravate your trigger points, try doing self-treatments before and after the activity. If you start getting sore or your symptoms get worse, decrease the frequency.

Take your balls with you on trips, since travel frequently aggravates trigger points. You may even want to keep some balls or a Backnobber at work.

Keep working on the muscle until it is no longer tender, even if your active symptoms have disappeared. Just because a trigger point isn't causing referred pain doesn't mean the trigger point is gone. It has probably just become latent, in which case it could easily be reactivated. If you leave your trigger points untreated or stop treatment too soon, it is more likely that the changes to your nervous system will be long-term or permanent, and that the pain will recur more easily. As your symptoms disappear, you may feel less motivated to do treatments or even forget to do them. Try not to let this happen. But if it does, the important thing is that you will know what to do if symptoms return.

General Guidelines for Stretches and Conditioning

It is very important to distinguish between stretching and conditioning exercises. With stretching, you gently lengthen the muscle fibers, whereas with conditioning exercises you're trying to strengthen the muscle. Doctors Travell and Simons (1983) found that active trigger points benefited from stretching but were usually aggravated by conditioning exercises in the early stages of treatment.

Often people start physical therapy and trigger point therapy at the same time, but this may be counterproductive, as physical therapy usually relies heavily on conditioning exercises unless the physical therapist is familiar with trigger points. In my experience, when the two are done concurrently in the initial stages of treatment, over half the time the person's condition either doesn't improve or actually gets worse. Usually you can start doing conditioning exercises after about two weeks of trigger point treatment and self-help work, but if your trigger points are still very irritable, you will need to wait until your symptoms improve. Meanwhile, learn the stretching exercises in this book. As long as you follow the guidelines, these do not need to be prescribed by a practitioner.

If you aren't sure whether an assigned activity is a stretch or a conditioning exercise, ask your practitioner. Also be sure to tell your practitioner all the activities, exercises, and stretches you're doing, because some of these could be contributing to activating your trigger points. I won't cover guidelines for conditioning exercises in depth here, since those exercises should be prescribed by a practitioner, who can also give you instructions for performing them safely and effectively.

Things to Avoid When Stretching and Conditioning

Avoid stretching when your muscles are tired or cold, and don't bounce on stretches. Friends may recommend conditioning exercises that worked for them, but you are a different person with a different set of symptoms, and you shouldn't do conditioning exercises prescribed for them, just as you wouldn't take their prescribed medications. If a conditioning exercise or stretch is aggravating your symptoms, stop doing it. Consult with your practitioner to determine why it is bothering you and how you should proceed.

When and How to Do Stretches and Conditioning

Do your stretches *after* treating your trigger points. If you have time to do only one thing, do the self-treatments and skip the stretches. Trigger point inactivation followed by stretching is more effective than trigger point inactivation alone, but stretching without prior inactivation can actually increase trigger point sensitivity (Edwards and Knowles 2003).

Stretch slowly, and only to the point of just getting a gentle stretch. Don't force it. If you stretch muscles too hard or too fast, you can aggravate trigger points. Hold each stretch for thirty to sixty seconds. There will be little benefit after thirty seconds, but stretching for longer won't harm you. You may repeat the stretch after releasing and breathing. For any type of repetitive exercise, breathe and rest between each repetition of the exercise.

If your stretches or conditioning exercises make you sore for more than one day, try again after the soreness has disappeared and reduce the number of repetitions. If you're still sore two days after the exercise or stretch, you may be doing it incorrectly or it might not be the right stretch for you and need to be eliminated or changed (Travell and Simons 1983).

General Guidelines for Muscle Care

In addition to deactivating your trigger points and doing your stretching, you need to take good care of your muscles. This will help prevent reactivation of old trigger points and the development of new ones.

Muscle Awareness

After treatments, gently use the muscle in a normal way, using its full range of motion, but avoid strenuous activities for at least one day or until the trigger points aren't so easily aggravated, whichever is longer. Go slowly and be gentle with yourself.

Rest and take frequent breaks from any given activity, and don't sit for too long in one position. Learn to avoid keeping your muscles in prolonged contractions, where you are holding them tense or using them in a sustained way. To increase blood flow and bring oxygen and nutrients to the muscles, they need to alternately constrict and relax, which normal, fairly frequent movement will accomplish. Notice where you hold tension and practice relaxing that area. Avoid cold drafts.

Lift with your knees bent and your back straight, holding the object you're lifting close to your chest. Don't lift something too heavy—ask for help. Never put the maximum load on a muscle. It's too easy to strain your muscles when you do this.

Exercise Programs

Before doing any type of exercise, warm up adequately. Tight, cold muscles are more prone to injury. As always, as with any exercise, avoid positions or activities that aggravate any medical condition. Swimming is generally a good exercise, and bicycling is easier on the body than running, but in both cases you must take care to avoid straining your trapezius and neck muscles. Any bike that allows you to sit more upright, such as a recumbent or stationary bicycle, is preferable to those that require you to lean over the handlebars.

When starting an exercise program, underestimate what you will be able to do, and err on the side of caution. Many people believe in the adage "No pain, no gain" and think that pushing through the pain will make them stronger. But this just aggravates existing problems and makes them harder to treat. Exercise should be comfortable. Alternate running with walking or, when lifting weights, rest between repetitions and use weights that aren't too heavy. If you tend to overdo things, you need to back off on your activities, then add them back in slowly with the guidance of your practitioner. Returning to activities too soon or doing them excessively will quickly erode your progress.

Gradually increase the duration, rate, and effort of any exercises in small increments that don't cause soreness or trigger point activation. Mild to moderate aerobic exercise is good for overall health and for preventing the recurrence of muscular problems. It's also great for reducing stress. People who exercise regularly are less likely to develop trigger points than those who exercise occasionally and overdo it. Just don't overdo it!

Conclusion

In this chapter, you've learned the basics of trigger point self-treatments, along with what to avoid when doing self-treatments. You've also learned some of the basics about how to stretch, and how to take care of your muscles to prevent reactivation of trigger points and the formation of new trigger points. The most important thing to remember is what not to do: don't overdo trigger point treatments, stretching, conditioning, or exercise programs. Review the guidelines in this chapter frequently in the beginning stages of treatment, and then review them periodically thereafter to ensure that you are performing the techniques properly.

The next chapter will help you identify which muscles may be causing your elbow, lower arm, wrist, or hand pain and other symptoms. It will also offer guidance on recording your symptoms and tracking your progress.

Chapter 9

Which Muscles Are Causing Your Pain?

The last chapter taught you *how* to treat trigger points; this chapter helps you find *where to look* for trigger points that are causing your particular set of symptoms.

Pain Map

To figure out which muscles to work on first, look at the Pain Map on pages 76 and 77. Find the area(s) where you feel your pain, and read the chapters identified by the numbers in parentheses. The muscles in the menus are listed from top to bottom in order of the most common muscles to refer pain to an area, but it may be different for you, so be sure to check all the chapters.

Look at the photos of referral patterns in each chapter, and try to find the ones that most closely match your pain pattern. Read the list of symptoms for each muscle. Do any of the referral patterns look familiar? Do any of the symptoms sound familiar? These are the ones you want to work on first.

Be sure to go back and read the rest of the chapters, because those trigger points may also play a role in your pain. You may need to work on all the listed muscles if you are not sure which muscle contains the trigger points that are causing your pain, or because trigger points in more than one muscle may be causing your pain.

You may wish to make copies of the blank body chart on page 76 and draw your symptom pattern on it with a colored marker. Then you can compare it with the pain referral pictures in chapters 10 through 30. Out to the side of each painful area, note your pain intensity on a scale of 1 to 10 and the percent of time you feel pain in that area, for example, "6.5/80%."

I recommend that you fill out a body chart at least a couple of times per week. Date them so you'll be able to keep them in order. This chronological record will come in handy in several ways: It will make it easier to discern which patterns fit your pain referral most closely. It will also help you recognize the factors that cause and perpetuate your symptoms by matching fluctuations in the level and frequency of your symptoms. And finally, it will allow you to track your progress (or lack thereof) and provide a historical record of any injuries. As your condition improves, you may forget how intense your symptoms were originally, and you may think you're not getting any better. The body charts will help prevent this frustration by graphically illustrating any reduction in the overall intensity or frequency of your pain and the extent of the area affected. You'll be able to see that you are improving, even if you have an occasional setback. One note: not everyone can accurately draw their pain location, due in part to lack of familiarity with anatomy, so take that possibility into consideration and check muscles with adjacent referral patterns just in case your drawing is inaccurate.

Muscle Chapters

Chapters 10 through 30 cover the major muscles commonly associated with elbow, lower arm, wrist, or hand pain and other symptoms. Most chapters contain an anatomical drawing of the muscle or muscles covered in that chapter. Photographs show the most common pain referral areas for each trigger point. The more solid black overlay area indicates the primary area of referral, which is almost always present, and the stippled area shows the most likely secondary areas of referral, which may or may not be present. The letter X marks spots where trigger points are most commonly found in conjunction with that referral pattern. There may be additional trigger points, so search the entire muscle.

The pain referral photographs in the muscle chapters show only the most common referral patterns; bear in mind that your referral pattern may be somewhat different or even completely different. Also, you may have overlapping referral patterns from trigger points in multiple muscles. These areas may be larger than the patterns common for individual muscles, so be sure to search for trigger points in all the muscles that refer pain to that area. Pain may be particularly intense in areas where you have overlapping pain referral.

In the following chapters, the information for each muscle includes lists of common symptoms and causes or perpetuators of trigger points. Again, these are only the most common; you may experience different symptoms, and your causes and perpetuating factors may be different. If you suspect trigger points in a certain muscle but don't see any causes listed that seem to apply to you, try to imagine whether anything in your life is similar to something on the list, in effect causing the same type of stress on the muscle. For example, perhaps you don't do any of the activities listed in the hand and finger extensor chapter (24), but you are a painter. Gripping a paint brush and making repetitive movements will cause trigger points to form in these muscles.

Most muscle chapters provide stretches for the muscle or muscles covered in that chapter. If you're seeing a practitioner, have them check to make sure you're performing the stretches properly. If your symptoms are getting worse, stop doing the self-help techniques and consult with your practitioner.

Conclusion

Once you've determined which two muscles most closely fit your pain pattern, start working on those. Over the next several weeks, start treating additional muscles. Periodically review the guidelines in chapter 8 to make sure you're doing the self-treatments properly. As you start to feel better, you'll develop a clearer picture of which trigger points in which muscles are causing your pain, and which perpetuating factors are reactivating your trigger points.

Arm Pain Map

The muscle names are followed by the chapter number

1. Scalene (20)
Supraspinatus (13)
Trapezius (10)
Triceps brachii (19)
Biceps brachii (23)

(Also Levator scapula,
Multifidi, Rhomboid, and
Splenius cervicis, which are
not addressed in this book.)

2. Scalene (20)
Latissimus dorsi (17)
Serratus posterior
    superior (15)
Infraspinatus (14)
Trapezius (10)
Serratus anterior (12)
Pectoralis major (11)

(Also Levator scapula,
Paraspinals, and Rhomboid,
which are not addressed in
this book.)

3. Scalene (20)
Supraspinatus (13)
Teres major (18)
Subscapularis (16)
Serratus posterior
    superior (15)
Latissimus dorsi (17)
Triceps brachii (19)
Trapezius (10)

(Also Deltoid, Levator
scapula, Teres minor, and
Iliocostalis thoracis, which
are not addressed in this
book)

4. Scalene (20)
Triceps brachii (19)
Subscapularis (16)
Supraspinatus (13)
Teres major (18)
Latissimus dorsi (17)
Serratus posterior
    superior (15)
Coracobrachialis (22)

(Also Deltoid and Teres
minor, which are not
addressed in this book.)

5. Triceps brachii (19)
Serratus posterior
    superior (15)

6. Supinator (25)
Hand / Finger extensors (24)
Triceps brachii /
    Anconeus (19)
Supraspinatus (13)

7. Triceps brachii (19)
Pectoralis major (11)
Pectoralis minor (21)
Serratus anterior (12)
Serratus posterior
    superior (15)

8. Triceps brachii (19)
Teres major (18)
Hand / Finger extensors (24)
Coracobrachialis (22)
Scalene (20)
Trapezius (10)

9. Infraspinatus (14)
Scalene (20)
Brachioradialis (24)
Supraspinatus (13)
Subclavius (11)

10. Latissimus dorsi (17)
Pectoralis major (11)
Pectoralis minor (21)
Serratus posterior
    superior (15)

11. Hand / Finger extensors (24)
Subscapularis (16)
Coracobrachialis (22)
Scalene (20)
Latissimus dorsi (17)
Serratus posterior
    superior (15)
First dorsal
    interosseous (30)
Trapezius (10)

12. Supinator (25)
Scalene (20)
Brachialis (28)
Infraspinatus (14)
Hand / Finger extensors (24)
Adductor / Opponens
    pollicis (29)
Subclavius (11)
First dorsal interosseous (30)
Flexor pollicis longus (27)

13. Finger extensor
    digitorum (24)
Hand interosseous (30)
Scalene (20)
Pectoralis major /
    Subclavius (11)
Pectoralis minor (21)
Latissimus dorsi (17)

14. Pectoralis major /
    Subclavius (11)
Pectoralis minor (21)
Scalene (20

(Also Sternocleidomastoid,
Sternalis, Intercostals /
Diaphragm, Iliocostalis
cervicis, and External
abdominal oblique, which
are not addressed in this
book.)

15. Infraspinatus (14)
Scalene (20)
Supraspinatus (13)
Pectoralis major /
    Subclavius (11)
Pectoralis minor (21)
Biceps brachii (23)
Coracobrachialis (22)
Latissimus dorsi (17)

(Also Deltoid and
Sternalis, which are not
addressed in this book.)

16. Scalene (20)
Infraspinatus (14)
Biceps brachii (23)
Brachialis (28)
Triceps brachii (19)
Supraspinatus (13)
Subclavius (11)

(Also Deltoid and
Sternalis, which are not
addressed in this book.)

17. Brachialis (28)
Biceps brachii (23)

18. Palmaris longus (26)
Pronator teres (27)
Serratus anterior (12)
Triceps brachii (19)

19. Hand / Finger flexors (27)
Opponens pollicis (29)
Pectoralis major (11)
Pectoralis minor (21)
Latissimus dorsi (17)
Palmaris longus (26)
Serratus anterior (12)

20. Flexores digitorum
    superficialis
    and profundus (27)
Hand interosseous (30)
Latissimus dorsi (17)
Serratus anterior (12)
Subclavius (11)

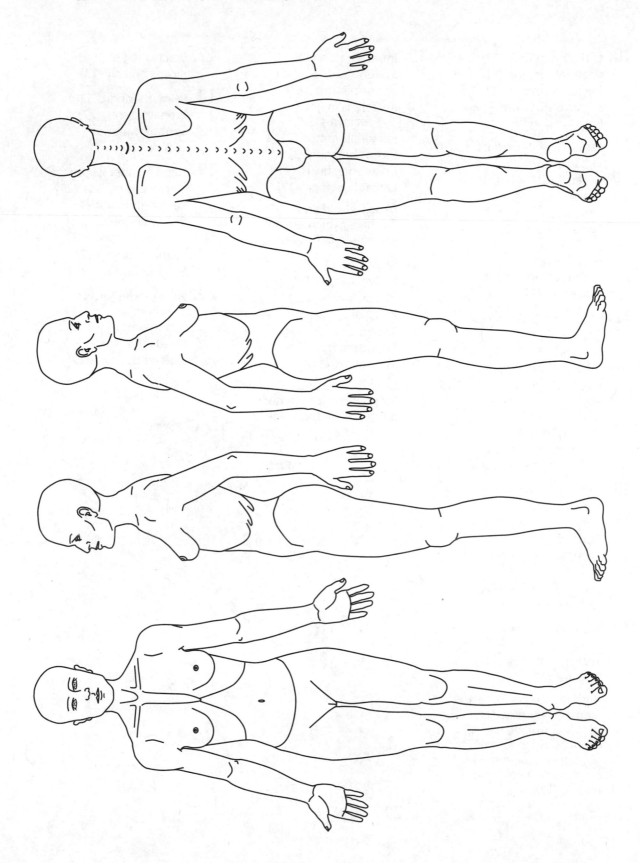

Chapter 10

Trapezius

The trapezius is a large, kite-shaped muscle covering much of the back and posterior neck. It commonly contains trigger points, and referred pain from these trigger points causes people to seek help more often than for trigger points in any other muscle.

Although referral down the arm from trapezius trigger points is relatively uncommon, and is caused only by trigger point #7, other trapezius trigger points can activate satellite trigger points in other muscles that subsequently cause referred pain down the arm. You may discover that you must treat the trapezius muscle first before you can gain lasting relief for your arm, elbow, wrist, and hand pain. If you suspect that trapezius trigger points are also causing neck and head pain, including headaches and migraines, see *Trigger Point Therapy for Headaches & Migraines: Your Self-Treatment Workbook for Pain Relief* (New Harbinger: 2008), since those areas are beyond the scope of this workbook.

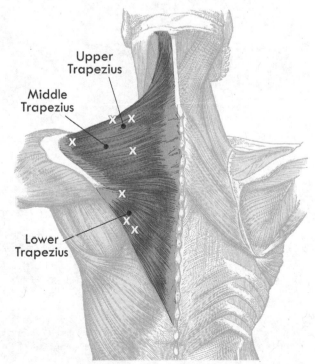

Common Symptoms

There are three main parts to the muscle: the upper, middle, and lower trapezius, and each part has its own actions and common symptoms.

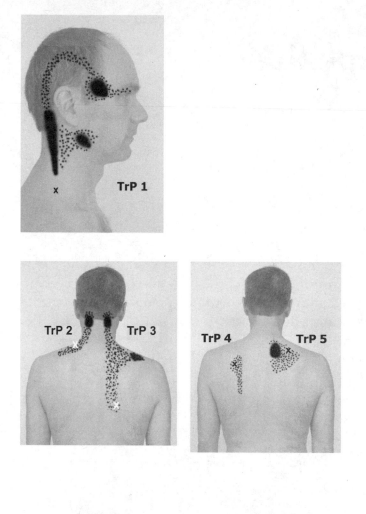

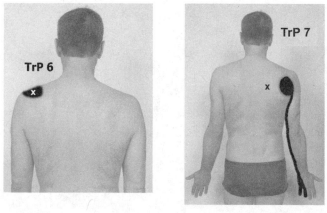

Upper Trapezius (trigger points #1 and #2)

- Trigger points refer pain to your temple, face, or jaw, and possibly behind your eye. You may get headaches over your temples and/ or tension headaches.

- You will likely have stiffness, limited range of motion, and/or severe pain in your neck, and won't be able to tolerate any weight on your shoulders.

- You may experience dizziness or vertigo (indicates simultaneous involvement of the sternocleidomastoid muscle, which is found in *Trigger Point Therapy for Headaches & Migraines: Your Self-Treatment Workbook for Pain Relief*).

Middle Trapezius (trigger points #5 and #6)

- Trigger points refer pain to the upper midback (trigger point #5 only).

- You may also experience superficial burning pain close to your spine (trigger point #5 only).

- Trigger points refer aching pain at the top of your shoulder near the joint (trigger point #6 only).

Lower Trapezius (trigger points #3, #4, and #7)

- Trigger points refer pain to the midback, neck, and/or upper shoulder region.

- You may experience headaches at the base of your skull (trigger point #3 only).

- You may possibly experience referred pain on the back of your shoulder blade, down the inside of your arm, and into the ring and little fingers—very similar to the referral pattern of the serratus posterior superior (trigger point #7 only).

- You may have deep aching and diffuse tenderness over the top of your shoulder (trigger point #3 only)

Possible Causes and Perpetuators

- Head-forward posture, tensing your shoulders, or turning your head to one side for long periods to have a conversation or to hear more clearly

- Poor posture at your desk such as cradling a phone between your ear and shoulder, sitting without a firm back support (sitting slumped), typing on a keyboard that's too high, and/or sitting in a chair without armrests or with armrests that are too high

- Bending over for extended periods (for example, if you are a dentist, hygienist, architect, draftsperson, or secretary, or have some other job that requires bending over a workspace)

- Sleeping on your front or back with your head rotated to the side for a long period

- Carrying a daypack or purse that is too heavy, or carrying it over one shoulder

- Wearing a bra with straps that are too tight (either the shoulder straps or the torso strap), or wearing a heavy coat

- Sports activities such as jogging, backpacking, bike riding, kayaking, tennis, and golfing

- Sewing on your lap with your arms unsupported

- Playing the violin

- Using a cane that is too long

- Getting a whiplash injury (from a car accident, falling on your head, or any sudden jerk of the head)

- Suffering from fatigue

- Having large breasts, one leg that is anatomically shorter than the other, sit bones that aren't level because one side is smaller, or short upper arms (which causes you to lean to one side to use armrests)

- Having tight pectoralis major muscles

Helpful Hints

When standing, you can put your hands in your pockets to help take the weight off of your trapezius muscles. If you wear a heavy coat, put shoulder pads in it.

If you backpack, try to put most of the weight on your hip strap. When biking, including using a stationary bike, sit as upright as possible by adjusting the handlebars. If you lift weights, use light weights and keep your head straight and in alignment with your shoulders. If you must use a cane, be sure it is the correct length, so that is does not elevate one shoulder.

Swimming provides good aerobic exercise, but you need to vary your strokes so that you don't stress the trapezius muscle. Turning your head to one side to breathe can aggravate the trapezius.

You may need to see a chiropractor or osteopathic physician to determine whether you have vertebrae out of alignment.

Self-Help Techniques

Applying Pressure

Trapezius Pressure

Lie faceup on a firm bed or the floor with your knees bent. Place a tennis ball or racquetball about one inch out to the side of your spine, starting at the top of your back, and hold pressure on that spot for eight seconds to one minute. Scoot a small distance to the next spot farther down the back in a line parallel to the spine, and again hold pressure on the spot. Continue working down all the way to the top of the pelvis in order to work on both the trapezius and the paraspinal muscles (the muscles that run in a lengthwise strip on either side of the spine). You may want to repeat this on a second line farther out from the spine, especially if you have a wide back or have trigger points farther out. *Do not do this directly on the spine, because you may injure yourself!* I recommend using one ball at a time, rather than using a ball on each side at the same time. By performing this technique lying down, as opposed to standing and leaning into a wall, you keep

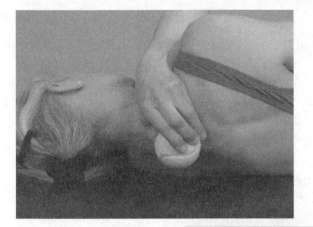
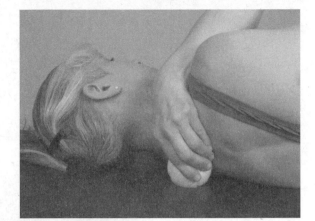

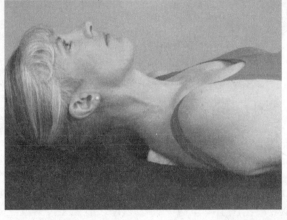

the muscles as passive as possible, since you aren't using them to hold you upright while you're applying pressure. The gradient in the photo at right marks the area you will want to work on.

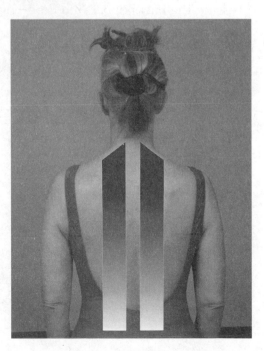

Upper Trapezius Pinch

Place your elbow and forearm on a surface high enough to support the weight of your arm. With the opposite hand, reach across your front and pinch the upper portion of the trapezius muscle. Be sure to stay on the meat of the muscle, and *don't dig your thumb into the depression directly above the collarbone, or you could injure delicate nerves and blood vessels.* You may need to tilt your head slightly toward the side you're working on to keep the muscle relaxed enough to be able to pinch it.

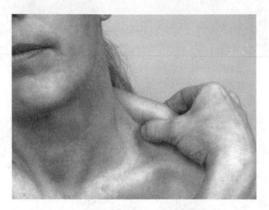

If you are at work or otherwise unable to lie on the floor, I recommend using a Backnobber, available from the Pressure Positive Company (see Resources). Note how both of my hands are pulling the Backnobber away from my body in the direction my fingers are pointing, rather than pressing the Backnobber into the front of my trunk to lever pressure onto my back.

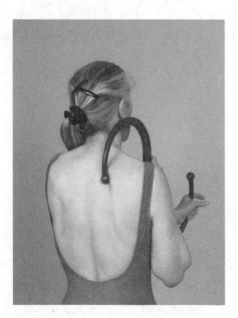

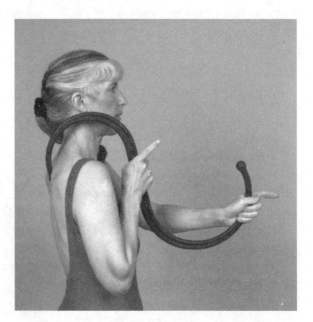

Stretches

Trapezius Stretch

This stretch benefits the middle and lower trapezius. Lie on your back with your arms at your sides, and then move your arms through the positions indicated in the photographs: Raise your arms so that your upper arms are perpendicular to the floor and your forearms are parallel to the floor, with your elbows bent at a 90-degree angle. Then, while still holding a 90-degree angle at your elbows, lower your hands so they touch the surface above your head. Next, extend your arms out straight above your head, palms up. Next, slide your upper arms down until they're perpendicular to your trunk and your elbows are again bent at a 90-degree angle, so that your forearms are parallel to your trunk. Last, bring your arms down to your sides and take two deep breaths. Repeat three to five times.

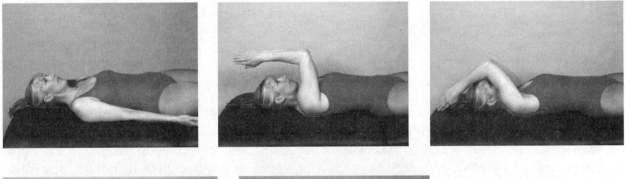

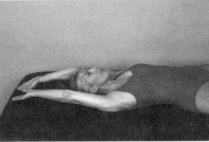
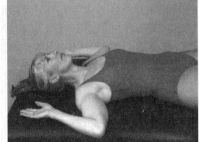

Pectoralis Stretch

The pectoralis stretch will also benefit the trapezius muscle; see chapter 11.

Other

Proper Posture

To learn proper posture and correct head-forward posture, see "Head-Forward Posture," chapter 5, Body Mechanics.

Also See

- Serratus posterior superior (chapter 15)
- Pectoralis major (chapter 11)
- Pectoralis minor (chapter 21)

Conclusion

Trigger points in the pectoralis major and pectoralis minor muscles may cause muscle tightness that subsequently puts a strain on the mid and upper back, keeping trapezius trigger points active. Trigger points in the serratus posterior superior have a referral pattern that is similar to trapezius trigger point #7. Although trapezius trigger points #1 through #6 do not directly cause arm or hand pain, they may activate trigger points in other muscles that *do* refer pain into the arm and hand.

For books that contain a list of other conditions that your medical health care provider may want to consider, see the Resources list.

Chapter 11

Pectoralis Major;
Subclavius

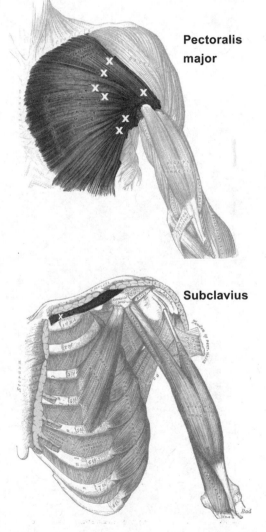

Pectoralis major

Subclavius

The pectoralis major muscle covers much of the chest, and it can cause shoulders to be rounded forward in a slumped-looking posture. The subclavius is located just below and tucked under the collarbone, running from the sternum (breastbone) to a point in the middle third of the collarbone.

Pectoralis major trigger points can mimic the symptoms of a heart attack, but can also be caused *by* a heart attack. Active trigger points in this muscle may also cause pain and a feeling of chest constriction that mimic *angina* (pain caused by reduced blood flow to an area of heart muscle). Chest pain caused by trigger points (rather than a heart attack or angina) is likely to be intermittent and intense when moving the upper arm. You may also experience pain at rest if the trigger points are very active. Since trigger points and angina and/or a heart attack can exist concurrently, *you will still need to undergo cardiac function tests even if you are able to relieve pain with trigger point self-help techniques; do not assume it is trigger points only!*

If you do have heart disease, pain from trigger points may reflexively diminish the size of the coronary arteries, thereby further increasing *myocardial ischemia* (a restriction of the blood supply to the heart), so relief of trigger points can increase cardiac circulation in addition to increasing comfort.

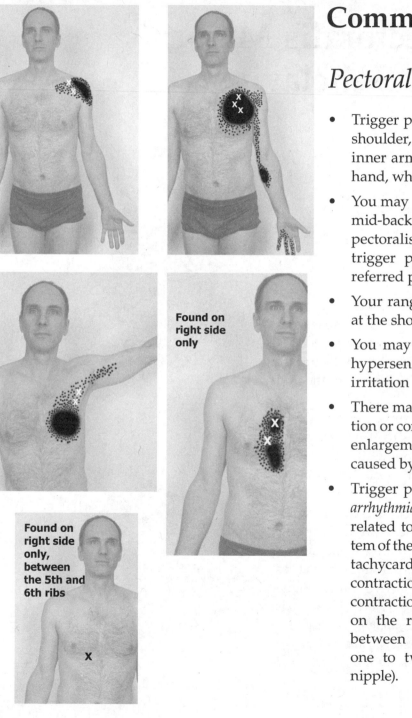

Found on right side only

Found on right side only, between the 5th and 6th ribs

Common Symptoms

Pectoralis Major

- Trigger points refer pain over the chest, shoulder, and breast, and down the inner arm, possibly all the way into the hand, which may disturb your sleep.

- You may experience pain referred to the mid-back area due to shortening of the pectoralis muscles, even if the pectoralis trigger points are latent (not causing referred pain of their own).

- Your range of motion may be restricted at the shoulder joint.

- You may experience breast tenderness, hypersensitivity of the nipple, and/or irritation caused by clothing.

- There may be a feeling of chest constriction or congestion in your breast (a slight enlargement, and a "doughy" feeling caused by impaired lymph drainage).

- Trigger points may cause *ectopic cardiac arrhythmias* (abnormal heart rhythms related to the electrical conduction system of the heart) such as supraventricular tachycardia, supraventricular premature contractions, or ventricular premature contraction (caused by a particular point on the right side of the trunk only, between the fifth and sixth rib, about one to two inches to the left of the nipple).

Subclavius

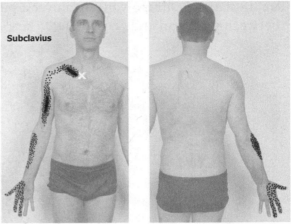

Subclavius

- Trigger points in the subclavius muscle can refer pain under the collarbone, down the front upper arm, down the outside of the lower arm, and into the thumb, index, and middle fingers. Shortening of the subclavius muscle by trigger points can contribute to vascular thoracic outlet syndrome by causing the clavicle to compress the subclavian artery and vein against the first rib.

Possible Causes and Perpetuators

- Slouching while sitting or standing, allowing your shoulders to round forward
- Heavy and/or sustained lifting, especially when reaching out in front, as with a chainsaw
- Bringing your arms together repetitively, as in using a pair of bush clippers
- Experiencing constant anxiety, probably resulting in holding your breath
- Having a heart attack, or undergoing open heart surgery where the incision was through the breastbone rather than through the ribs
- Immobilizing your arm in a cast or sling
- Exposing your muscles to cold air when they are fatigued

Helpful Hints

Get a good pair of custom orthotics that will shift your weight slightly to the balls of your feet. This will shift your head back over your shoulders, bring your shoulders back, and restore normal cervical and lumbar curves. Get a chair with a good lumbar support, and buy a portable lumbar support for your car or any seat (including your couch at home) that doesn't have adequate lumbar support. You may wish to even take a lumbar support to the movie theater, or when traveling for use on airplanes and in rental cars. If you sit in bleachers or go on picnics, get some type of back support like a Crazy Creek Chair (found in sporting goods stores) so you have at least some kind of support.

Crossing your arms in front of you shortens the pectoralis major muscle, so try to use armrests at the height of your elbows. If you must perform work that requires you to lift or hold tools out in front, take frequent breaks—but try to avoid the activity all together. When lying on your unaffected side, drape your arm over a pillow. When lying on the affected side, tuck a pillow between your arm and chest/belly to keep your arm out at a 90-degree angle.

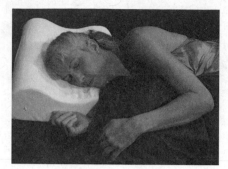

If your bras leave indentations on the skin, they are too tight and need to be replaced.

Self-Help Techniques

Applying Pressure

Pectoralis Pressure

Lie facedown, with your arm next to your side. Place a ball above your breast area. Be sure to work all the way out to the armpit. You may need to shift your weight a little to that side as you work out toward the armpit. You may also try hanging your arm over the side of your bed, if it is high enough to allow your arm to dangle. If you are large-breasted, you may find it easier to place the ball on the end of a couch arm or wall and lean into it, but be sure to keep your arm relaxed.

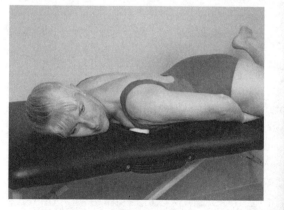

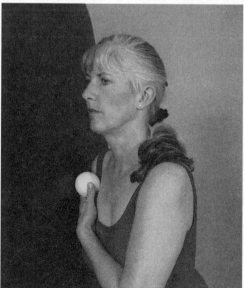

Subclavius Pressure

Much of the subclavius muscle is under the collarbone, so you must lean forward, allowing your arm to dangle, which moves your collarbone away from your trunk. With your opposite hand, press under the collarbone with your fingers, working from close to the breastbone (sternum) to a few inches out toward the shoulder.

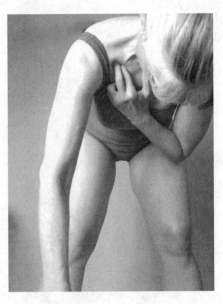

Stretches

Pectoralis Stretch

Stand in a doorway and place your forearm along the doorframe, including your elbow. With the foot of the same side placed about one step forward, rotate your body gently away from the side you are stretching.

Move your forearm up to about a 45-degree angle and repeat.

Bring the forearm down below the first position and repeat. These positions will stretch different parts of the muscle.

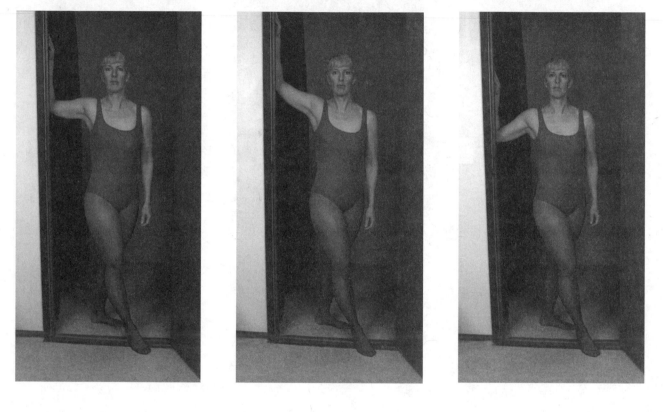

Also See

- Scalenes (chapter 20)
- Coracobrachialis (chapter 22)
- Serratus anterior (chapter 12)
- Trapezius (chapter 10)
- Infraspinatus (chapter 14)
- Subscapularis (chapter 16)
- Latissimus dorsi (chapter 17)
- Teres major (chapter 18)

Conclusion

The trapezius muscle (chapter 10) may become painful after relieving pectoralis major trigger points. The coracobrachialis (chapter 22), scalenes (chapter 20), trapezius, and serratus anterior (chapter 12) muscles will tend to develop satellite trigger points. The anterior deltoid, sternalis, sternocleidomastoid, and rhomboid muscles will also tend to develop satellite trigger points, but since they don't directly cause elbow, lower arm, wrist, or hand pain, they are not addressed in this book. See the Resources section for books and other resources for self-treatment of muscles not covered in this book.

If you have been diagnosed with thoracic outlet syndrome, also search for trigger points in the latissimus dorsi (chapter 17), teres major (chapter 18), scalenes (chapter 20), and subscapularis (chapter 16) muscles, since trigger points in those muscles may mimic thoracic outlet syndrome.

For books that contain a list of other conditions that your medical health care provider may want to consider, see the Resources list.

Chapter 12

Serratus Anterior

The serratus anterior fibers cover much of the side of the trunk, running from several ribs to the edge of the shoulder blade (*scapula*), functioning to move the scapula, and preventing it from "winging" away from the trunk, in addition to assisting in breathing. In my experience, it rarely gets treated by bodyworkers.

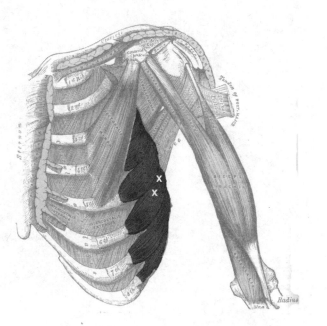

Common Symptoms

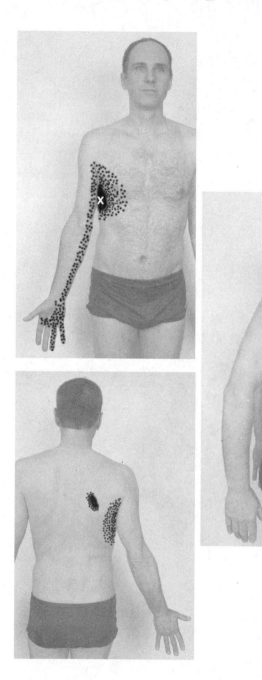

- Trigger points refer pain primarily on the side of the chest underneath the armpit, and to a spot in the midback next to the lower end of the shoulder blade. They may possibly refer pain down the inside of the arm and into the palm, and ring and little fingers.

- You may have pain with deep breathing, and shortness of breath to the extent you may feel you cannot get enough air or finish a sentence without stopping to breathe. You may refer to it as a "stitch in the side."

- You may have difficulty lying on that side or getting comfortable at night, and possibly have tender breasts.

- You may have "winging" of the shoulder blade, where the top of the shoulder blade is pulled away from the trunk, and your shoulders may be rounded forward.

- The nerves that supply the serratus anterior can be entrapped by the scalene muscles.

Possible Causes and Perpetuators

- Muscle strain from athletic activities such as push-ups, running very fast or for long periods, or forceful swimming, as in the butterfly stroke
- Lifting heavy objects overhead
- Coughing forcefully
- Having high levels of anxiety
- Having a heart attack

Helpful Hints

If you have a chronic cough, you will need to address the underlying causes. If you are unable to eliminate the cough, you will need to expel phlegm by clearing the throat or using a cough expectorant, or use a cough suppressant. Acupuncture and herbs are very successful at treating coughs and phlegm.

Avoid push-ups and chin-ups, and overhead lifting. Lie on the unaffected side, and drape your opposite arm over a pillow.

Learn proper breathing techniques. Taking a few *deep* slow breaths may be helpful. Treat anxiety with acupuncture, herbs, homeopathy, and/or counseling. Reduce stressful situations.

You may need to see a chiropractor or osteopathic physician to be evaluated for mid-thoracic vertebrae being out of alignment.

Self-Help Techniques

Applying Pressure

Serratus Anterior Pressure

Lie on the unaffected side, and use the fingers of that side to apply pressure to the other side of the rib cage below the armpit. It is a fairly large area, so check toward your breast and back toward your shoulder blade, and almost to the bottom of your rib cage.

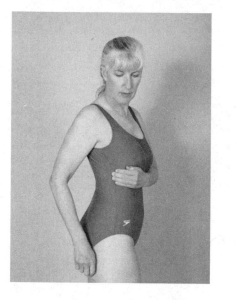
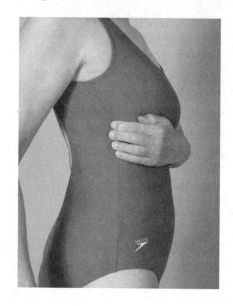

Stretches

Pectoralis Stretch

The pectoralis stretch will also benefit the serratus anterior muscle; see chapter 11. The middle and lower positions will stretch the serratus anterior.

Serratus Anterior Stretch

Hang your arm over the back of a chair, and rotate your trunk away from the side you are stretching.

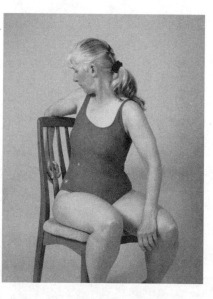

Also See

- Latissimus dorsi (chapter 17)
- Scalenes (chapter 20)
- Trapezius (chapter 10)
- Serratus posterior superior (chapter 15)

Conclusion

Also search the trapezius (chapter 10) muscle, since some of the trigger points can cause similar pain symptoms, and/or may have related trigger points. The serratus posterior superior (chapter 15) may also harbor trigger points simultaneously. Trigger points in the serratus anterior may cause trigger points in the latissimus dorsi (chapter 17) and scalene (chapter 20) muscles, because they are also used for breathing.

The rhomboid and paraspinal muscles can also cause similar pain symptoms, and/or may have related trigger points. Trigger points in the serratus anterior may also cause trigger points in the sternocleidomastoid muscles, because they are also used for breathing. Other muscles that can cause a "stitch in the side" are the diaphragm or the external abdominal oblique. Since trigger points in these muscles don't directly cause elbow, lower arm, wrist, or hand pain, they are not addressed in this book. See the Resources section for books and other resources for self-treatment of muscles not covered in this book.

For books that contain a list of other conditions that your medical health care provider may want to consider, see the Resources list.

Chapter 13

Supraspinatus

This is one of the muscles forming the "rotator cuff," along with the infraspinatus, teres minor, and subscapularis. Unfortunately, all too often pain felt in the shoulder area is given a diagnosis of a *rotator cuff injury* without investigating the cause of the pain. A rotator cuff tear must be diagnosed with an MRI, and it is helpful to know which muscle or muscles contain the tear. Pain from a rotator cuff tear is severe and usually exhibits a limited arc of motion.

Pain is more often due to trigger points in one of those areas, and may also be present even if a tear is confirmed, especially if tightness in the muscle from trigger points contributed to the overload that led to the tear. Subdeltoid bursitis, rotator cuff tears, and supraspinatus trigger points may all cause tenderness where the tendons of the rotator cuff muscles attach at the shoulder joint, but only trigger points will cause spot tenderness in the midportion of the supraspinatus muscle. Any of these conditions can occur simultaneously with trigger points, or trigger points can get misdiagnosed as one of these conditions.

Trigger points in the supraspinatus muscle can also cause referred pain down the arm, and are rarely addressed and treated.

Common Symptoms

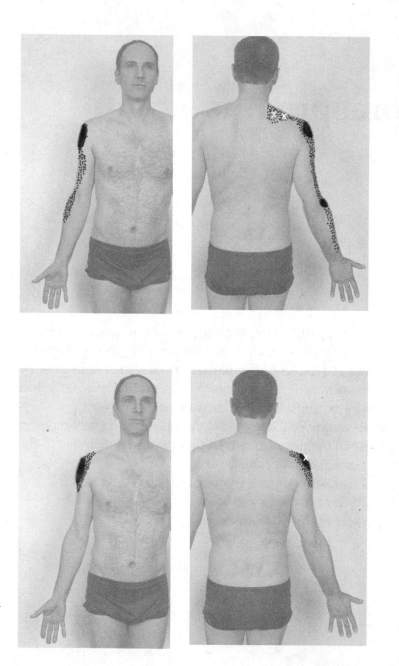

- Trigger points can cause a deep ache in the shoulder area, mainly around the outside of the upper end of the upper arm. Referred pain may be felt strongly in the elbow, and/or run down the outside of the arm, sometimes all the way to the wrist.

- Pain is worse with lifting the arm, and there is a dull ache when resting the arm. The shoulder may make clicking or snapping sounds, probably due to the tight muscle interfering with the normal glide of the shoulder joint.

- Moderately restricted range of motion is more noticeable when reaching toward the head or with sports. You may be unable to reach behind your back and touch the opposite shoulder blade with your fingers.

- You may possibly experience stiffness and aching when in bed.

Possible Causes and Perpetuators

- Carrying heavy objects with your arm at your side, such as a heavy purse, laptop, briefcase, or luggage
- Walking a dog that pulls on the leash
- Lifting a heavy object to or above shoulder height

Helpful Hints

Don't lift items overhead or hold your arms out or up continuously. Get luggage with wheels or ask for help with carrying it. Use a daypack instead of a briefcase or heavy purse, or get a shoulder strap that you can wear diagonally across your torso.

Get a head halter for a dog that pulls. It will prevent most breeds from pulling.

You may need to see a chiropractor or osteopathic physician to be evaluated for a C5 or C6 vertebra out of alignment in the neck.

Self-Help Techniques

Applying Pressure

Supraspinatus Pressure

Stand in a doorway and place a tennis ball in the groove in the doorjamb, and continue to hold onto the ball with your opposite hand. Bend over at about 90 degrees, and *be sure to let your head go completely limp!* Lean into the ball with however much pressure you want to apply. Still holding onto the ball with your opposite hand and continuing to keep your head fully relaxed, work spots across the top of the shoulder. Avoid this technique if you have balance problems or high blood pressure, or if there is any other reason it is uncomfortable for you.

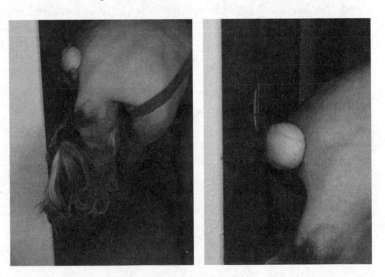

Stretches

Infraspinatus Stretch

The infraspinatus stretch will also benefit the supraspinatus; see chapter 14. If there is any suspicion of a tear in one of the rotator cuff muscles, *do not stretch this muscle until a tear is ruled out by an MRI. Do only the pressure self-work described above prior to getting an MRI, or if a tear is confirmed.*

Also See

- Infraspinatus (chapter 14)
- Trapezius (chapter 10)
- Latissimus dorsi (chapter 17)
- Subscapularis (chapter 16)

Conclusion

Be sure to also search for trigger points in the infraspinatus (chapter 14), trapezius (chapter 10), and subscapularis (chapter 16) muscles, since they are nearly always also involved. You may also need to work on the latissimus dorsi muscle (chapter 17).

The deltoid muscle tends to develop satellite trigger points, but since these trigger points don't directly cause elbow, lower arm, wrist, or hand pain, they are not addressed in this book. See the Resources section for books and other resources for self-treatment of muscles not covered in this book.

For books that contain a list of other conditions that your medical health care provider may want to consider, see the Resources list.

Chapter 14

Infraspinatus

One of the four muscles forming the "rotator cuff," the infraspinatus muscle lies over the back of the shoulder blade, or scapula. Trigger points in this area are becoming increasingly common as people spend more time on computers, especially on the side used as the "mouse arm."

The other three muscles comprising the rotator cuff are the supraspinatus, teres minor, and subscapularis. Unfortunately, all too often pain felt in the shoulder area is given a diagnosis of a "rotator cuff injury" without investigating the cause of the pain, so they are rarely addressed and treated. A rotator cuff tear must be diagnosed with an MRI, and it is helpful to know which muscle or muscles contain the tear. Pain is more often due to trigger points in one of those areas, and may also be present even if a tear is confirmed, especially if tightness in the muscle from trigger points contributed to the overload that led to the tear.

Trigger points in the infraspinatus muscle can also cause referred pain down the arm.

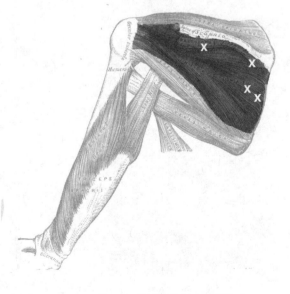

Back of shoulder blade

Common Symptoms

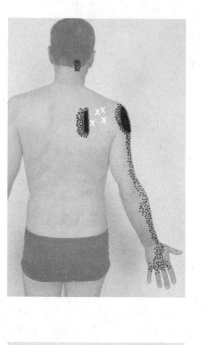

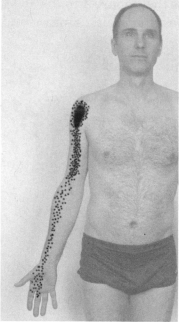

- Trigger points refer pain felt deep in the front of the shoulder and deep within the joint. Pain can be referred into the forearm and occasionally all the way to the fingers, or even into the base of the skull.

- Occasionally pain will be referred to the midback area over the rhomboid muscles, and sometimes this will activate and perpetuate the lower trapezius trigger points, which must be inactivated before infraspinatus trigger points can be inactivated.

- You may possibly experience referred pain when sleeping on either the affected or opposite side at night, which disrupts your sleep.

- Your arm may "fall asleep" at night, and sometimes even during the day (this is a defining symptom of trigger points in the infraspinatus).

- You probably have difficulty reaching behind your back or sometimes raising your arm to your head in front.

- You probably experience loss of mobility, fatigue of the area around the shoulder joint, and/or "weakness" of your grip. If you play tennis, you will likely have a lack of power with tennis strokes.

- You may experience *hyperhydrosis* (excessive sweating at times when you would not normally sweat, that is, not due to exercising or extreme heat) in the area of pain referral, but this is relatively uncommon.

- Entrapment of the suprascapular nerve can cause shoulder pain and atrophy of the infraspinatus.

Possible Causes and Perpetuators

- Pulling a sled, wagon, or person behind you, or reaching behind you to get something off a nightstand

- Sports activities such as hard tennis serves or pushing yourself with ski poles

- A sudden overload of the muscle by arresting yourself from a fall or trying to hold on to something heavy

- Anything that requires you to hold your arms out in front of you for extended periods with your arms not well supported, such as computer use (especially your "mouse arm"), kayaking, driving, or tennis

Helpful Hints

Avoid activities that overload the muscles, such as holding your arms over your head while styling your hair, or reaching backward to reach items on a bedside table.

Apply heat packs to the muscle at bedtime for fifteen to twenty minutes. As always with the application of heat, be sure to rest the pack on the muscle rather than lying on the heat pack, which can cut off needed circulation and cause burns. Lie on the side that isn't bothering you, and drape your affected arm over a pillow for support.

Modify or replace your misfitting furniture. See chapter 5 for a description of an ergonomically correct workstation. This is probably the most important factor to address to relieve infraspinatus trigger points.

Self-Help Techniques

Applying Pressure

Infraspinatus Pressure

This is one of the more challenging muscles to learn, as people nearly always initially work in the rhomboid area (in the midback), thinking they have succeeded in finding the infraspinatus muscle since the rhomboid area is almost always also tender.

Lie on the affected side with your arm out at a 90-degree angle, and thoroughly search the back of the shoulder blade. If you are lying on your back, you are probably getting too far in toward the spine. Try reaching under your arm and locating the muscle with your fingertips first, as with most people this is where their fingers will reach. Be sure to work all the way out to your armpit, and then you will know you are getting the right area. Most people will need to do this on the bed with a fairly soft ball, since this muscle is usually quite tender.

If lying on it is too painful, an alternative is to put a ball in a long sock and dangle the sock over your shoulder, and lean against a wall or couch with however much pressure is

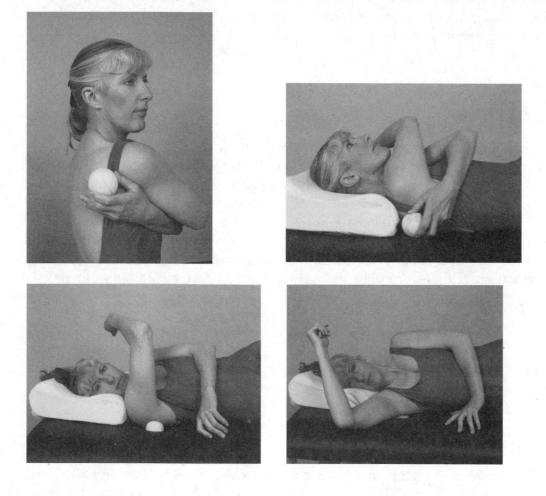

comfortable. Remember, you will need to angle your body at about a 45-degree angle from the wall or couch, or you will get in too close to the spine and miss the infraspinatus. The affected arm should be totally relaxed. When the tenderness decreases, start performing your self-work on the bed, since this is the preferred position.

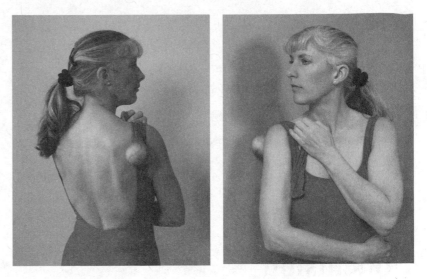

Stretches

Infraspinatus Stretch

Stretch by grasping the affected arm above the elbow, and bring your arm across your chest.

Then, put your arm behind your back, and use the opposite hand to grasp at the wrist, and gently pull on the affected arm. You can do this in a warm shower to help facilitate the stretch.

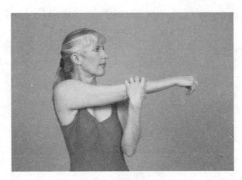

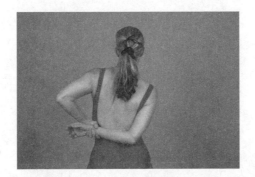

Also See

- Supraspinatus (chapter 13)

- Pectoralis major (chapter 11)

- Teres major (chapter 18)

- Latissimus dorsi (chapter 17)

- Biceps brachii (chapter 23)

- Subscapularis (chapter 16)

Conclusion

Also search for trigger points in the supraspinatus (chapter 13), teres major (chapter 18), pectoralis major (chapter 11), latissimus dorsi (chapter 17), subscapularis (chapter 16), and biceps brachii (chapter 23), since some of these muscles are usually also involved. The teres minor and deltoid muscles may also develop trigger points that need to be treated at some point, but since trigger points in these muscles don't directly cause elbow, lower arm, wrist, or hand pain, they are not addressed in this book. See the Resources section for books and other resources for self-treatment of muscles not covered in this book.

If you have been unsuccessfully treated for bicipital tendinitis or scapulohumeral syndrome, search the infraspinatus (14), biceps (23), pectoralis major (11), and pectoralis minor (21) muscles for trigger points. For books that contain a list of several other conditions that your medical health care provider may want to consider, see the Resources list.

Chapter 15

Serratus Posterior Superior

This muscle frequently contains trigger points, and often gets missed by massage therapists because the shoulder blade needs to be moved out of the way in order to access the most common trigger point. Placing the arm over the side of the massage table moves the shoulder blade forward and exposes the trigger point. The self-help technique below contains instructions for moving your shoulder blade out of the way.

Common Symptoms

- Trigger points refer pain over the shoulder blade (often a deep ache), down the back of the arm, and into the little finger.

- Occasionally pain may be felt in the upper chest area.

- Pain may be increased by lifting objects out in front of you, or by lying on the affected side, due to the shoulder blade pressing on the trigger points.

- You may experience referred numbness into your hand.

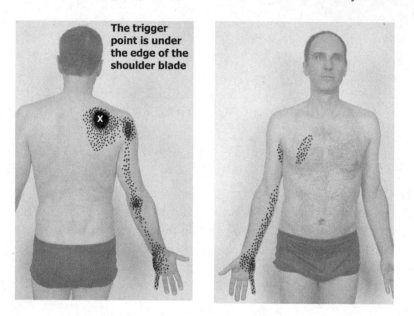

The trigger point is under the edge of the shoulder blade

Possible Causes and Perpetuators

- Writing at a high desk or table, or reaching far forward frequently

- The shoulder blade compressing the muscle against the underlying rib, or severe spinal scoliosis

- Coughing, asthma, emphysema, and improper breathing techniques

Helpful Hints

Use a lumbar support at work, home, and while traveling. Make sure your desk or table is at a proper height, and that your arms are well-supported. See the section on spinal problems in chapter 5.

Learn to breathe properly; see pectoralis minor (chapter 21).

Self-Help Techniques

Applying Pressure

Serratus Posterior Superior Pressure

This one is a little tricky to get with the ball. You *must* hold your arm across your chest while lying on the ball, and be sure to get all the way up next to the top of the inner edge of the shoulder blade. It will also likely be tender lower, so you may think you have gotten the trigger point, but have actually missed it. If you don't hold your arm across your chest, your arm will drop down a little bit, and the shoulder blade will cover the trigger point. You may want to seek the help of a massage therapist to make sure you are getting this point.

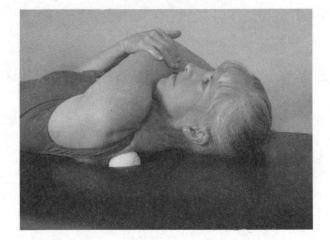

Also See

- Scalenes (chapter 20)

Conclusion

Also search the scalene muscles (chapter 20), since trigger points in that muscle may cause trigger points in the serratus posterior superior, or occasionally vice versa. The rhomboid, iliocostalis thoracis, longissimus thoracis, and multifidi muscles may contain related trigger points, but since trigger points in these muscles don't directly cause elbow, lower arm, wrist, or hand pain, they are not addressed in this book. See the Resources section for books and other resources for self-treatment of muscles not covered in this book.

Referred numbness from serratus posterior superior trigger points into the hand may be mistaken for a C8/T1 nerve root irritation, so be sure to check for trigger points if you have been given this diagnosis. You may need to see a chiropractor or osteopathic physician for evaluation of a T1 vertebra out of alignment near the base of the neck. There will usually be tenderness over the vertebra if this is the case.

For books that contain a list of several other conditions that your medical health care provider may want to consider, see the Resources list.

Chapter 16

Subscapularis

This is one of four muscles that form the "rotator cuff," along with the supraspinatus, infraspinatus, and teres minor. Unfortunately, all too often pain felt in the shoulder area is given a diagnosis of a "rotator cuff injury" without investigating the cause of the pain. A rotator cuff tear must be diagnosed with an MRI, and it is helpful to know which muscle or muscles contain the tear. Pain is more often due to trigger points in one of those areas, and may also be present even if a tear is confirmed, especially if tightness in the muscle from trigger points contributed to the overload that led to the tear.

For a discussion of thoracic outlet syndrome, see chapter 3, since the subscapularis may be involved.

Trigger points in the subscapularis muscle primarily cause extremely painful restriction of motion, and the diagnosis of "frozen shoulder" or "adhesive capsulitis" is often used. This is a general term used to describe shoulder pain and restriction of movement, and is usually not a specific diagnosis of what is *actually going on physiologically* in the shoulder girdle. As symptoms get worse, you can't lift your arm above shoulder level, and you can't reach across your chest. Pain is constant whether using or resting your arm, but it is worse with movement and worse at night. The other muscles that typically

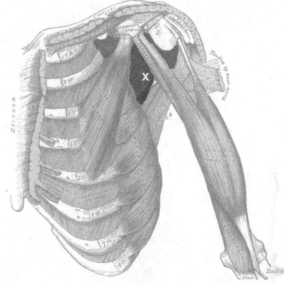

View from the front of the body. The muscle is on the front of the shoulder blade.

get involved with the subscapularis in a frozen shoulder are the pectoralis major, latissimus dorsi, and teres major.

Sometimes thickened tissues are found in the shoulder girdle area in the muscles, the synovial capsule, bursa, or ligaments, but the problem still likely began with trigger points in the subscapularis muscle. In fact, trigger points in the subscapularis can cause blood vessels to constrict, causing a decrease in oxygen to the tissue, and subsequently actually *form* fibrous, or thickened, tissues in adjacent muscles and lead to adhesive capsulitis. Those trigger points and any trigger points in the surrounding affected muscles must be treated in order for therapy to be effective. Simons, Travell, and Simons, in chapters 18 and 26 of *The Upper Half of the Body* (1999), have a lengthy discussion of the use of the term "frozen shoulder" and treatment for the shoulder girdle area. I highly encourage you to read this if you are diagnosed with adhesive capsulitis or frozen shoulder, and perhaps share the information with your doctor and therapist. Often this condition is treated too aggressively in the initial stages, causing increased pain and involvement of additional muscles.

Acupuncture is very effective in treating pain and restricted motion in the shoulder area, usually coupled with use of a "TDP" heating lamp (TDP is an acronym for the Chinese name of the far-infrared technology the lamp uses) and/or use of *moxa*—an herb burned or sprayed over the local area. Chinese herbal formulas can be very effective in treating frozen shoulder quickly. If you decide to take Chinese herbs, I highly recommend having the herbs prescribed and supervised by someone trained in Chinese medicine. I definitely recommend trying alternative techniques before considering surgery, unless an MRI has determined that muscles, tendons, or ligaments are seriously torn or detached, in which case surgery is necessary.

Common Symptoms

- Trigger points refer severe pain primarily over the back of the deltoid area, but may also refer over the shoulder blade and down the triceps area, and possibly cause a straplike area of referred pain and tenderness around the wrist, which is worse on the back side.

- You may experience an inability to reach backward with the arm at shoulder level, as when throwing a ball, and restricted range of motion, often severely limited as the condition progresses.

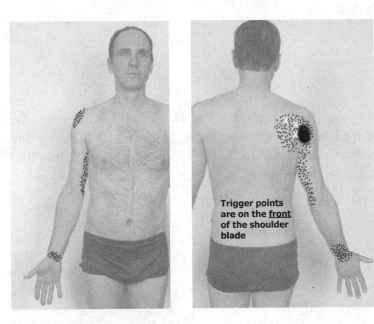

Trigger points are on the <u>front</u> of the shoulder blade

Possible Causes and Perpetuators

- Sudden trauma, such as reaching back to stop yourself from falling, catching a falling object or an object thrown to you, dislocating your shoulder, breaking the upper arm, or tearing the shoulder joint capsule

- Overuse of muscles that aren't accustomed to repetitive motions, such as swimming the crawl stroke or pitching a ball, or repeated forceful overhead lifting, as when swinging a child up and down

- Sitting with slumped posture

- Long-term immobilization, such as in a cast and shoulder splint

Helpful Hints

When you sleep on the affected side or your back, use a pillow between your trunk and upper arm to keep your arm out at a 90-degree angle. When the affected side is toward the ceiling, drape your arm over a pillow. When sitting, move your arm frequently, resting it on the back of the couch or car seat, or an armrest. When standing, hook your thumb in your belt. See chapter 5 for more information on body mechanics and proper furniture.

Self-Help Techniques

Applying Pressure

Subscapularis Pressure

The subscapularis is located on the anterior (front) surface of the shoulder blade, between the shoulder blade and the rib cage, making it difficult to access with finger pressure. Treating this muscle will require the assistance of a therapist of some kind, as the subscapularis is difficult to access on your own, but you can still do the stretch below.

Stretches

Subscapularis Stretch

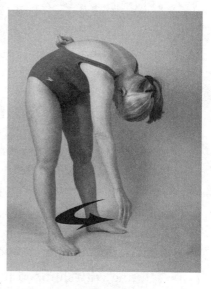

Lean over with your arm hanging down, and swing your arm widely in a clockwise direction for the left arm, and counterclockwise for the right arm. Be sure to keep your head totally relaxed.

You may also stretch this muscle by resting your arm across the back of a car seat or couch, reaching your arm up and behind your head, or reaching toward the ceiling.

Pectoralis Stretch

Stretching the pectoralis muscles will help treat the subscapularis muscle; see chapter 11.

Exercises

See chapter 5 for an exercise for postural retraining.

Also See

- Pectoralis major (chapter 11)
- Teres major (chapter 18)
- Latissimus dorsi (chapter 17)
- Triceps brachii (satellite trigger points – chapter 19)
- Supraspinatus (chapter 13)
- Infraspinatus (chapter 14)

Conclusion

Related trigger points may also be found in pectoralis major (chapter 11), the teres major (chapter 18), latissimus dorsi (chapter 17), supraspinatus (chapter 13), and infraspinatus (chapter 14), so be sure to search for trigger points in those muscles. The triceps brachii (chapter 19) may contain satellite trigger points. The deltoid muscle may also contain satellite trigger points, but since they don't directly cause elbow, lower arm, wrist, or hand pain, they are not addressed in this book. See the Resources section for books and other resources for self-treatment of muscles not covered in this book.

Pain from subscapularis trigger points can either mimic or occur concurrently with several other conditions. For books that contain a list of several other conditions that your medical health care provider may want to consider, see the Resources list.

Chapter 17

Latissimus Dorsi

The latissimus dorsi muscle is an often-overlooked source of trigger point referral, primarily because there are many other muscles that cause symptom referral in the same area. If you have pain in this area and working on other muscles has given no or only temporary relief, be sure to check this muscle for tenderness. Of its two trigger points, the one under the armpit is the more common culprit.

This muscle may get involved in "frozen shoulder." See the subscapularis muscle (chapter 16) for a discussion of that condition.

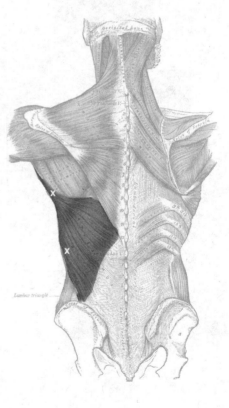

Common Symptoms

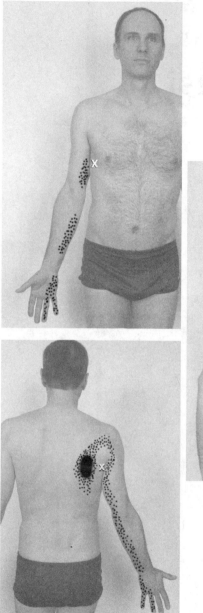

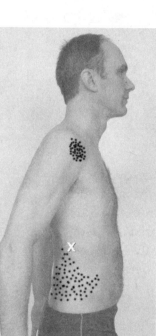

- The primary area of trigger point referral is under and adjacent to the bottom of the shoulder blade, with a constant, dull ache.

- Pain can sometimes travel down the arm and into the ring and little fingers.

- There is a less common trigger point on the side, above the waist, that refers pain to the front of the shoulder and sometimes just above the hip area.

- Initially pain may *only* be caused by lifting a heavy object in front of you, and not felt at rest. It is difficult to obtain relief by moving around, and pain will be worse as you reach up and out with a heavy object in your hands.

- If you are unable to identify any particular activity that aggravates midback pain, latissimus dorsi trigger points may be your culprit.

Possible Causes and Perpetuators

- Carrying boxes or other heavy objects in front of you, working with a heavy chainsaw at shoulder level, or throwing heavy bags of laundry or other objects repeatedly

- Weight lifting or pulling weights down overhead, or hanging from a swing or rope

- Weeding a garden

- Sports activities such as swimming aggressively with the butterfly stroke or throwing a baseball

- Wearing a bra with a tight strap around your chest

Helpful Hints

Avoid reaching up and above to hold or retrieve objects. Use a foot stool or stepladder if necessary. If you must pull down on something, keep your upper arm at your side.

At night, avoid drawing your arm tightly into your body. Instead, try to keep your elbow out away from your body. You may try putting a pillow next to your trunk to help with this.

Wear bras that fit properly. If you see elastic marks on your skin after you take your bra off, the straps are too tight. Jogging bras work great for medium or small-breasted women. Have the salesperson help you find a bra that fits properly—many of them really know their products.

Self-Help Techniques

Applying Pressure

Latissimus Dorsi Pressure

With the arm of the affected side resting on the back of a couch, use your opposite hand to reach under your armpit and pinch an area about one inch below the armpit. Be sure to pinch as close to the rib cage as possible, rather than just pinching a fold of skin. Pressing with the fingers may be more effective for some people, and will be effective for reaching the lower trigger points.

You may also try lying on a tennis or racquet ball if the muscle is not too tender. Try lying on the bed, with your arm out straight above your head. The tender spot will likely be just below the armpit.

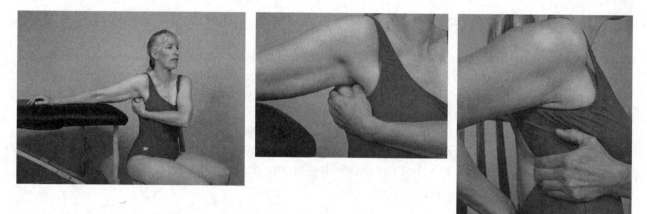

Stretches

Follow the stretches with a hot pack applied for fifteen to twenty minutes. Lay the hot pack on your body as opposed to lying on the hot pack, which can cut off needed circulation and can cause burns.

Latissimus Dorsi Stretch

Wrap the hand of the affected side behind your head, and touch your fingers to your opposite ear if possible, and reach even further forward if you are not forcing the stretch.

Pectoralis Stretch

Stretching the pectoralis muscles will help treat the latissimus dorsi; see chapter 11.

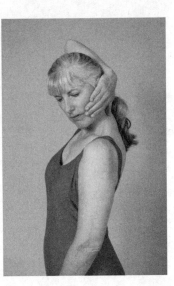

Also See

- Teres major (chapter 18)
- Triceps brachii (satellite trigger points – chapter 19)
- Subscapularis (chapter16)
- Serratus anterior (chapter 12)
- Serratus posterior superior (chapter 15)
- Hand and finger flexors (satellite trigger points – chapter 27)
- Trapezius (lower portion, satellite trigger points – chapter 10)

Conclusion

Search for trigger points in the serratus posterior superior (chapter 15), since pain referral from that muscle can cause trigger points in the latissimus dorsi. Also search for trigger points in the teres major (chapter 18) and triceps brachii (chapter 19) muscles, since they often will develop trigger points concurrently with the latissimus dorsi.

Referred pain from the latissimus dorsi and other muscles can be misdiagnosed as thoracic outlet syndrome. See the scalenes chapter (chapter 3) for a discussion of that syndrome and the other muscles that may be involved.

You may need to see a chiropractor or osteopathic physician to be evaluated for innominate dysfunction or misalignment of any of the vertebrae between and including T7 in the mid back and L4 in the lumbar area. The head of the humerus (upper arm bone) may need to be checked for its position in the shoulder joint. For books that contain a list of several other conditions that your medical health care provider may want to consider, see the Resources list.

Chapter 18

Teres Major

The teres major forms the back "wall" of the armpit, along with the latissimus dorsi muscle.

If the posterior deltoid, teres minor, and subscapularis also develop trigger points, range of motion can be greatly restricted and the shoulder area can become very painful, resulting in "frozen shoulder." See the subscapularis muscle, chapter 16, for a discussion of frozen shoulder. Referred pain from the teres major can be misdiagnosed as thoracic outlet syndrome. See chapter 3 for a discussion of that syndrome and the other muscles that may be involved.

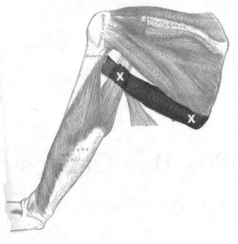

View from the back of the body.

Common Symptoms

- Trigger points refer pain primarily to the outside and back of the shoulder and over the back of the upper arm, and sometimes over the back of the forearm. Pain is usually felt when using the arm out in front, or when reaching forward and up.

- There may be a slight restriction in range of motion when reaching overhead, but for most people not likely a noticeable amount.

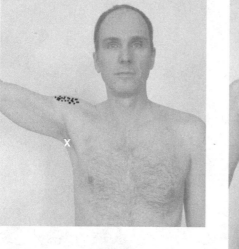
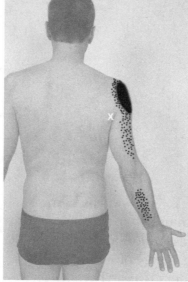

Possible Causes and Perpetuators

- Any activity that requires sustained resistance, such as driving a car that is hard to steer

- Activities such as lifting weights overhead, giving a massage using your elbows, or dancing with a partner who forces your arms into position

Helpful Hints

Avoid strenuous activities that aggravate trigger points in the teres major (such as lifting weights overhead) until self-help techniques have lessened the pain substantially. Be sure your car is easy to steer, or that any activity you perform on a regular basis is modified until it no longer causes trigger point activation.

At night, drape your affected arm over a pillow.

Self-Help Techniques

Applying Pressure

Teres Major Pressure

Lie on your side and extend your arm so that it is sticking straight up above your head, and rest on a tennis ball to apply pressure. Remember, the teres major forms the back "wall" of the armpit, so be sure you are applying pressure to that area.

You may also rest the arm on the back of a couch or adjacent chair and pinch the muscle in between your thumb and fingers.

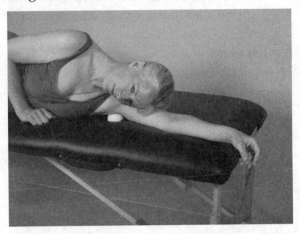

Stretches

Triceps Stretch

The triceps brachii stretch will benefit the teres major muscle; see chapter 19.

Also See

- Latissimus dorsi (chapter 17)
- Triceps brachii (chapter 19)
- Subscapularis (chapter 16)

Conclusion

Commonly, trigger points will also be found in the latissimus dorsi (chapter 17) and triceps brachii (chapter 19) muscles. If the posterior deltoid, teres minor, and subscapularis (chapter 16) also become involved and result in a painful frozen shoulder, then you will also need to search for trigger points in and work on those muscles. Relieving teres major trigger points may release tightness in the rhomboid muscle that may have developed because of a tight teres major pulling on the midback area. Since the deltoid, teres minor, and rhomboid muscles don't directly cause elbow, lower arm, wrist, or hand pain, they are not addressed in this book. See the Resources section for books and other resources for self-treatment of muscles not covered in this book.

Referred pain from the teres major and other muscles can be misdiagnosed as thoracic outlet syndrome. See chapter 3 for a discussion of that syndrome and the other muscles that may be involved.

For books that contain a list of several other conditions that your medical health care provider may want to consider, see the Resources list.

Chapter 19

Triceps Brachii;
Anconeus

Trigger points in these muscles are very common, and unfortunately, also commonly overlooked by practitioners. The anconeus and all heads of the triceps brachii are used to straighten your arm at the elbow. The head of the triceps that crosses the shoulder joint is also used to move the upper arm. All of these play a major role in elbow pain; see chapter 3 for a discussion on tennis elbow.

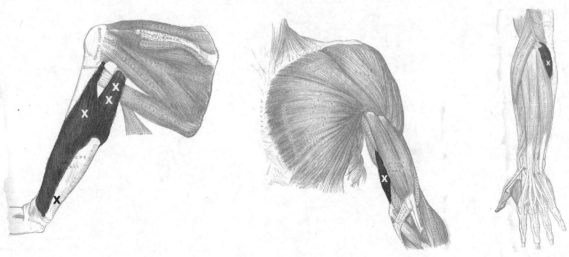

View from the from back of the body   **View from the front of the body**   **Back of the forearm**

Common Symptoms

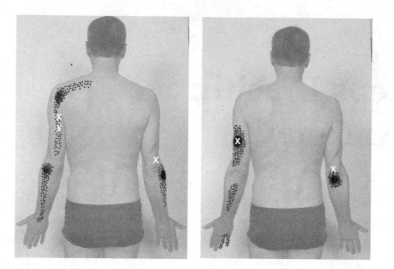

- See the pictures for all the various pain referral patterns. Pain around the elbow is one of the most common referral patterns, and often causes and perpetuates trigger points in adjacent muscles.

- You may possibly experience pain with pressing or tapping on one of the bony parts of the elbow. Pain from some trigger points may be activated only during certain sports that require full forceful extension at the elbow, such as tennis and golf.

- If the triceps entraps the radial nerve, you may get tingling and numbness over the back of the lower forearm, wrist, and hand to the middle finger.

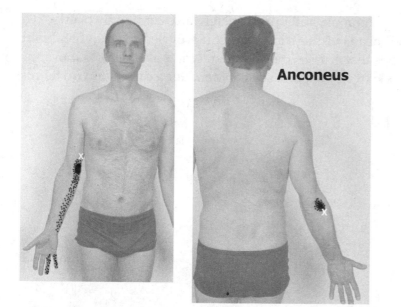

Anconeus

Possible Causes and Perpetuators

- Participating in sports that can cause strains, such as tennis, golf, or excessive conditioning (for example, push-ups, chin-ups)
- Driving for long periods, especially with excessive manual gear shifting
- Hand-sewing without elbow support, or using a computer without proper arm supports
- Working in a profession that requires a lot of pressure with the arms, such as with massage therapy, or repetitively pressing bound books onto a copy machine
- Having short upper arms
- Using forearm crutches, or a cane that is too long

Helpful Hints

Keep your upper arms by your side as much as possible when typing, writing, reading, and sewing, and use armrests of a proper height whenever possible; you shouldn't have to lean to the side—the arms should be at the height of your elbow.

Use a lighter tennis racquet or shorten the grip. Avoid chin-ups and push-ups.

Start using forearm crutches gradually, if at all possible.

Self-Help Techniques

Applying Pressure

Triceps and Anconeus Pressure

Lie on your side with your arm extended above your head. If you want less pressure, put your head on a pillow *behind* your upper arm. If you want more pressure, rest your head *on* your upper arm. Using a tennis or racquet ball, rest your upper arm on the ball, working all the way from the back of your shoulder down to your elbow. Be sure to get the front and back edges of the muscle too, by rotating the arm a little in both directions, since this muscle covers the entire back of the upper arm and trigger points can be found throughout the muscle. You may also pinch this muscle.

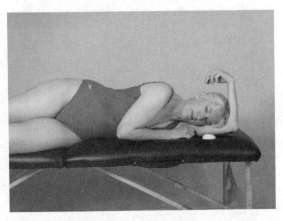

Stretches

Triceps Stretch

Standing sideways to the wall, place your elbow on the wall above your head with your forearm bent and your hand behind your head. Lean slightly into the wall to get a gentle stretch for both the triceps and teres major.

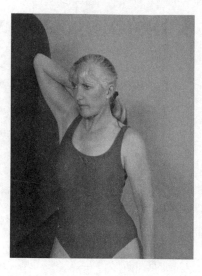

Also See

- Biceps brachii (chapter 23)

- Brachialis (chapter 28)

- Latissimus dorsi (chapter 17)

- Teres major (chapter 18)

- Supinator (chapter 25)

- Hand extensors, brachioradialis (extensor carpi radialis longus, brachioradialis – chapter 24)

- Serratus posterior superior (chapter 15)

Conclusion

You may also need to work on the latissimus dorsi (chapter 17), teres major (chapter 18), supinator (chapter 25), extensors carpi radialis longus and brachioradialis (chapter 24), and serratus posterior superior (chapter 15) muscles to obtain complete relief.

For books that contain a list of several conditions that your medical health care provider may want to consider, see the Resources list.

Chapter 20

Scalenes
(Scalenus Anterior, Medius, and Posterior)

Scalene trigger points are a major contributor to back, shoulder, and arm pain, and are commonly overlooked. They also contribute to headaches when combined with trigger points in neck and chewing muscles.

Thoracic outlet syndrome is commonly caused by scalene trigger points. Due to lack of information on the part of health care practitioners, these usually remain undiagnosed and untreated. See chapter 3 for a discussion of this condition and a list of trigger points in other muscles that can cause similar referral patterns.

The symptoms of carpal tunnel syndrome can also be mimicked by scalene trigger points. Carpel tunnel syndrome (or *pseudo*-carpal tunnel syndrome) may occur in conjunction with thoracic outlet syndrome. If you have been diagnosed with carpel tunnel syndrome, it is worth checking for trigger points in the scalenes (the scalenus anterior, medius, and posterior), pectoralis minor, and muscles in the forearm. See chapter 4 for a discussion of this condition and related trigger points.

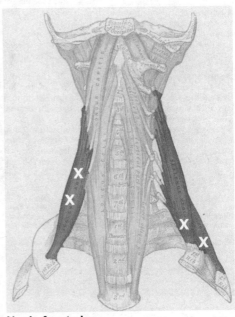

Neck, front view

Common Symptoms

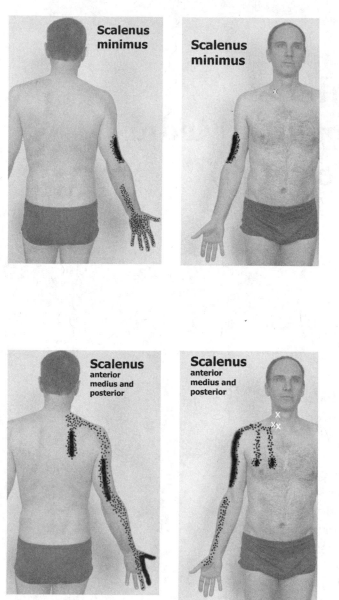

- Trigger points refer pain to the chest and midback, and/or over the outside, back, and front of the arm and into the wrist and hand. Pain on the left side may be mistaken for angina.

- Pain may disturb your sleep, but it is relieved by sleeping in a sitting position or propped up.

- You may be able to reproduce pain by turning your head to the side, and then moving your chin down toward the shoulder. You may be able to relieve pain by putting the back of your forearm across your forehead and moving your elbow forward (which moves your collarbone away from the scalene muscle).

- You likely experience minimal restriction of range of motion when rotating your head, but greater restriction when bending it to the side.

- You may drop items unexpectedly, and possibly experience finger stiffness. You may also have perceived (but not actual) numbness of the thumb, and tingling. If your arm has been amputated, you may have phantom limb pain.

- A tight scalene muscle may elevate your first rib, leading to compressed nerves, arteries, veins, and lymph ducts, causing numbness, tingling, and loss of sensation in your fourth and fifth fingers and the side of your hand. You may also have stiffness and swelling in your fingers and the back of your hand, which is worse in the morning.

Possible Causes and Perpetuators

- Activities such as horse handling or riding, playing tug-of-war, hauling ropes while sailing, competitive swimming, or playing some musical instruments

- Poor body mechanics while pulling or lifting, especially with your hands at waist level; carrying awkwardly large objects; or sitting with an arm rest that is too high or too low

- Injuries, such as whiplash from a car accident or falling on your head; limping; or surgical removal of a heavy breast

- Sleeping with your head and neck lower than the rest of your body, as when the bed is tilted

- Trigger points in the sternocleidomastoid or levator scapula muscles

- Improper breathing techniques, or coughing due to an acute or chronic illness

- Skeletal asymmetries such as an anatomically shorter leg, a small hemipelvis (either the right or left half of the pelvis), an extra rib at the top (a "cervical rib"), or the loss of an arm

- Spinal problems such as scoliosis (the spine isn't straight), or pain from a bulging or herniated cervical disc, which may linger even after surgery

Helpful Hints

Avoid carrying packages in front of your body, or pulling hard on anything.

When seated, make sure your elbow is resting on something, and that you are sitting straight rather than tilted to the side, no matter what your activity. Make sure that you have good lighting from behind when you read, so your head isn't turned to the side. If you have difficulty hearing and tend to turn to one side to hear better, turn your entire body to the side, or get a hearing aid if possible.

Use a headset for the phone rather than holding it to your ear or cradling it between your ear and shoulder. When using a computer, make sure the monitor is straight ahead and at eye level. Your elbows and forearms should rest comfortably on the chair armrests, neither too short so that you lean to one side, nor too tall so that they hike up your shoulders. See chapter 5 for a complete discussion of workstation ergonomics.

Don't read in bed. When getting up from a lying position, roll onto your side first, and when rolling over in bed, keep your head on the pillow rather than lifting it. Elevate the head of your bed two to three inches to provide mild traction at night. Multiple pillows will not provide the same effect, and will probably cause more pain. You should get a good nonspringy pillow that provides support for the cervical spine and keeps the spine in alignment. A chiropractor's office usually will carry well-designed pillows.

Apply heat to the front of your neck before bedtime. Keep cold drafts off of your neck by using a scarf or neck gaiter.

Learn to breathe properly; see chapter 21 for instructions. Eliminate the causes of coughing by treating the underlying illness as quickly as possible; see "Acute or Chronic Infections" chapter 7 for more information.

If you have a short leg or small hemipelvis (even as little as 3/8 inch difference), you will need to get fitted by a specialist for lifts to compensate, or it is unlikely you will be able to resolve scalene trigger points. Even if you have an extra cervical rib, relieving the scalene trigger points may be enough to eliminate symptoms.

Self-Help Techniques

Applying Pressure

Scalene Pressure

I do not teach patients to apply pressure to this muscle, due to all the major nerves and arteries in the front of the neck. You will need to go to a trained practitioner such as a massage therapist.

Stretches

If you are doing the pectoralis stretch, until the scalenes have improved, do only the top two positions and not the bottom one. If you have an extra cervical rib, do only the top position.

Side-Bending Neck Stretch

Lie face up, with the hand of the side you are stretching pinned under your butt. Put your opposite hand over the top of your head, and, looking straight at the ceiling, pull your head gently toward your shoulder, then release and take a deep breath. Repeat with your head turned slightly toward the left, and again with your head turned slightly toward the right. This will stretch different parts of the muscle. Do the other side the same way. You may repeat this stretch a few more times. You may apply heat prior to this stretch.

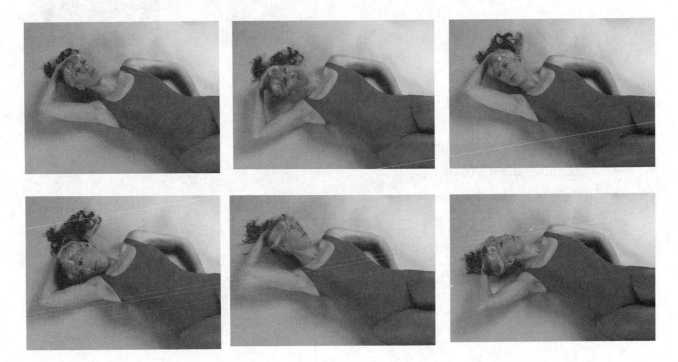

Scalenes Stretch

While sitting up, rotate your head all the way to one side, then bring your chin down. Return to the forward position and take a deep breath. Repeat on the opposite side. You may do this up to four times in each direction.

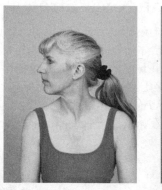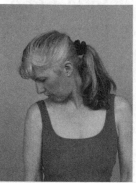

Also See

- Trapezius (upper portion – chapter 10)
- Pectoralis major, subclavius (both muscles – chapter 11)
- Pectoralis minor (chapter 21)
- Latissimus dorsi (chapter 17)
- Teres major (chapter 18)
- Subscapularis (chapter 16)
- Triceps brachii (satellite trigger points – chapter 19)
- Brachialis (chapter 28)
- Brachioradialis and hand extensors (extensors carpi radialis, extensor carpi ulnaris, and extensor digitorum – chapter 24)

Conclusion

Trigger points in the sternocleidomastoid or levator scapula muscles may cause trigger points to form in the scalene muscles, there may be related trigger points in the posterior neck, and scalene trigger points may cause satellite trigger points to form in the deltoid muscle, but since they don't directly cause elbow, lower arm, wrist, or hand pain, these other muscles are not addressed in this book. See the Resources section for books and other resources for self-treatment of muscles not covered in this book.

You may need to see a doctor to check for nerve root irritation at the C-5–C-6 vertebrae in the neck, because the pain pattern can be very similar to scalene trigger points, or they may be found together. You may need to see a chiropractor or osteopathic physician to be evaluated for T1, C4, C5, and C6 vertebral misalignments in the neck and at the base of the neck, or elevation of the first rib.

For books that contain a list of several other conditions that your medical health care provider may want to consider, see the Resources list.

Chapter 21

Pectoralis Minor

Trigger points are common in the pectoralis minor muscle, and can cause pseudo–carpal tunnel syndrome due to a pectoralis minor entrapment (see below.) See chapter 4 for an additional discussion about this condition, and to discover other trigger points that may be misdiagnosed as carpal tunnel syndrome.

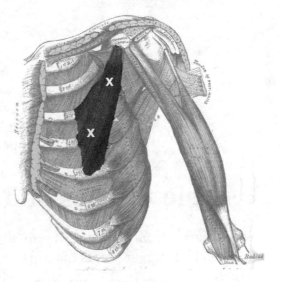

Common Symptoms

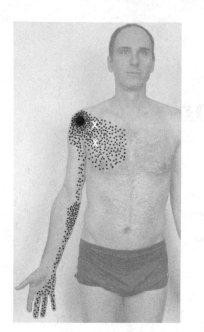

- Trigger points mainly refer pain over the front of the shoulder, and sometimes over the chest and/or down the inside of the arm into the middle, ring, and little fingers.

- Your shoulders will typically be rounded forward, and your range of motion will likely be restricted when reaching forward and upward, or reaching backward with your arm at shoulder level.

- Symptoms may mimic angina, and/or you may have difficulty in taking a deep breath.

- A pectoralis minor entrapment (pinching the axillary artery and the brachial plexus nerve) can be misdiagnosed as carpal tunnel syndrome, and will not be resolved by carpal tunnel surgery. Entrapment of the brachial plexus nerve causes numbness and uncomfortable sensations of the ring and little fingers, back of the hand, outside of the forearm, and palm side of the thumb, index, and middle fingers. Shortening of the pectoralis minor muscle fibers as a result of trigger points may lead to coracoid pressure syndrome, arm pain, and weakness of muscles in the midback in the areas of the lower portion of the trapezius and rhomboid muscles.

Possible Causes and Perpetuators

- Referral from scalene or pectoralis major trigger points, or angina pain that causes satellite trigger points to form in the pectoralis major muscle

- Weakness of the lower portion of the trapezius muscle

- Poor posture, especially when seated

- Receiving a trauma (such as getting fractured ribs), firing a rifle with the butt on the chest instead of the front of the shoulder, getting a whiplash injury, or open-heart surgery that was conducted through the breastbone (sternum) rather than through the ribs

- Gardening or other activities that require forceful movement of the arm at the shoulder girdle

- Coughing or improper breathing
- Wearing constricting gear, such as a daypack or backpack without a chest strap, allowing the shoulder straps to compress the muscle, or using crutches

Helpful Hints

Modify or replace your misfitting furniture; see chapter 5 for a discussion of proper ergonomics and posture.

Be sure to use a pack with proper shoulder padding and a chest strap to distribute weight away from the armpit area. Avoid bras that compress the pectoralis minor muscle. Try to find one with a wider shoulder strap or a padded strap. Use crutches properly by supporting your weight on your hands, not your armpits.

Self-Help Techniques

Applying Pressure

Pectoralis Pressure

See the pectoralis major muscle (chapter 11) for this pressure technique.

Stretches

Pectoralis Stretch

See the pectoralis major muscle (chapter 11) for this stretch.

Other

Learn to Breathe Properly

Place one hand on your chest and the other on your belly. When you inhale, both hands should rise. As you exhale, both hands should fall. You need to train yourself to notice when you're breathing only into your chest and make sure you start breathing into your belly.

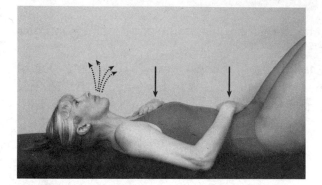 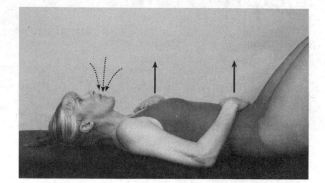

Also See

- Pectoralis major (chapter 11)
- Scalenes (chapter 20)

Conclusion

Search for trigger points in the pectoralis major (chapter 11) and scalene muscles (chapter 20), since they will keep trigger points in the pectoralis minor activated. The sternocleidomastoid and sternalis muscles may contain related trigger points, and the deltoid muscle may contain satellite trigger points, but since they don't directly cause elbow, lower arm, wrist, or hand pain, they are not addressed in this book. See the Resources section for books and other resources for self-treatment of muscles not covered in this book.

You may need to see a chiropractor or osteopathic physician to be evaluated for elevation of the third, fourth, and fifth ribs. For books that contain a list of several other conditions that your medical health care provider may want to consider, see the Resources list.

Chapter 22

Coracobrachialis

The coracobrachialis muscle is on the front of the shoulder, in the crease between the trunk and the upper arm. Not everyone has this muscle. This is a good one to check if you have already searched for and inactivated trigger points in the deltoid, pectoralis major, latissimus dorsi, teres major, supraspinatus, triceps, and biceps muscles, and have not gotten total relief.

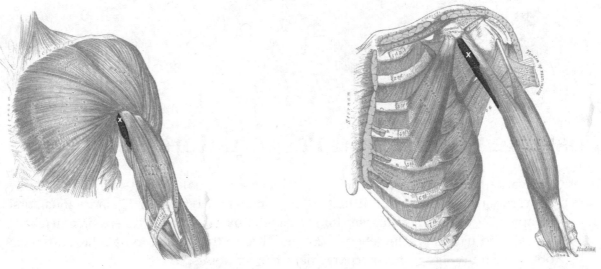

View from front of body

Common Symptoms

- Trigger points refer pain to the anterior deltoid (on the front of the upper arm), over the triceps on the back of the upper arm, down the back of the lower arm, and sometimes into the back of the hand and middle finger.

- When placing your affected arm in the small of your back, it is difficult to get your hand past the spine without pain, whereas normally you should be able to touch the other arm with your fingers. If by chance *only* the coracobrachialis is involved, you will feel pain when reaching forward and up above your ear while your arm is straight, and range of motion will be restricted.

- An entrapment of the musculocutaneous nerve may cause atrophy of the biceps muscle and reduced sensation on the back of the lower arm.

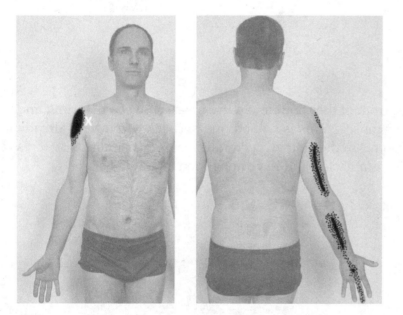

Possible Causes and Perpetuators

- Activation of trigger points in the coracobrachialis usually occurs *only* as a satellite area from trigger points in the deltoid, pectoralis major (chapter 11), latissimus dorsi (chapter 17), teres major (chapter 18), supraspinatus (chapter 13), triceps brachii (chapter 19), and biceps brachii (chapter 23) muscles, so these need to be relieved first to obtain lasting relief from coracobrachialis trigger points.

Helpful Hints

When lifting, hold objects close to your body, with your palms faceup as much as possible.

Self-Help Techniques

Applying Pressure

Coracobrachialis Pressure

Using the hand of the unaffected side, wrap your fingers around the deltoid muscle, and with your thumb knuckle bent, dig your thumb into the front of your shoulder on the outside of the crease, pressing toward the bone in the upper arm. Some of my patients have found they prefer to use something like a golf ball or a pressure gadget of some kind (often sold in massage stores or catalogs).

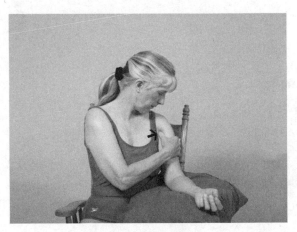

Stretches

Warm the area with moist heat before performing stretches.

Pectoralis Stretch

Use the pectoralis stretch, lower hand position; see chapter 11.

Doorjamb Stretch

See chapter 23, biceps brachii muscle, for this stretch

Couch Stretch

Stretch the muscle by placing your arm over the back of a couch and rotating the shoulder forward.

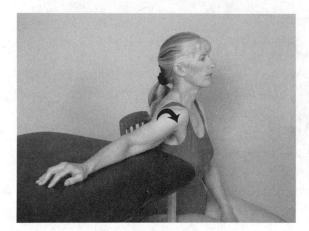

Also See

- Supraspinatus (chapter 13)
- Triceps brachii (chapter 19)
- Biceps brachii (chapter 23)
- Pectoralis major (chapter 11)
- Teres major (chapter 18)
- Latissimus dorsi (chapter 17)

Conclusion

There may be related trigger points in the deltoid muscle, but since they don't directly cause elbow, lower arm, wrist, or hand pain, they are not addressed in this book. See the Resources section for books and other resources for self-treatment of muscles not covered in this book.

For books that contain a list of several other conditions that your medical health care provider may want to consider, see the Resources list.

Chapter 23

Biceps Brachii

Though trigger points in the biceps are less common than many of the other trigger points that cause elbow, lower arm, wrist, or hand pain, they can develop due to particular repetitive motion injuries, or if you try to catch yourself during a fall (see below).

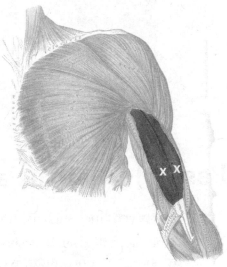

View from front

Common Symptoms

- Trigger points are typically found in the mid-to-lower part of the muscle, and commonly refer superficial achy pain over the front of the upper arm and front of the shoulder. You may possibly feel an ache or soreness over the upper trapezius (top of the shoulder) or in the crease opposite the elbow.

- You probably experience weakness and pain with raising your hand above your head with your elbow bent.

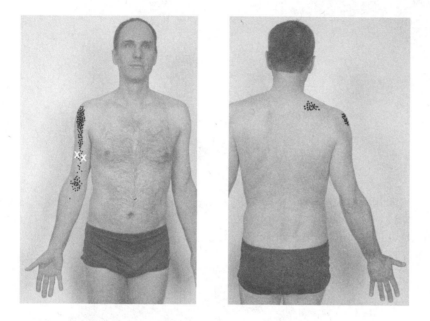

Possible Causes and Perpetuators

- Sports activities such as throwing a ball, or playing basketball or tennis
- Other activities such as shoveling snow, using a screwdriver for a long period, playing the violin or guitar, writing (with either a pen or a keyboard), or lifting heavy objects with your palms facing upward and/or with your arms extended forward
- Trying to catch yourself from falling
- Trigger points in the infraspinatus muscle can cause satellite trigger points in the biceps brachii.

Helpful Hints

Carry items either with your palms down, or in a daypack.

At night, be sure not to draw your arm tightly into your body. Instead, try to keep the elbow out from the body. You may try putting a pillow in the crook of your elbow to help with this.

Self-Help Techniques

Applying Pressure

Biceps Pressure

With the opposite hand, either pinch the biceps between the thumb and next two fingers, or just use your thumb to apply pressure.

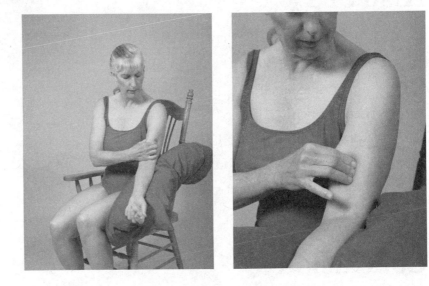

Stretches

Doorjamb Stretch

The doorjamb stretch will help treat the biceps muscle. Stand in a doorway with your arm straightened at slightly more than 90 degrees, with your palm on the doorjamb and the thumb pointing down. Put your foot of the same side one step forward, and rotate your body gently away from your hand. As you rotate your shoulder forward and down, you'll feel the stretch move into the front portion of the deltoid and the coracobrachialis, and the biceps.

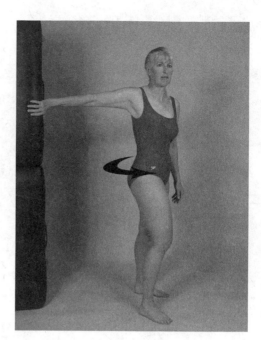

Also See

- Infraspinatus (chapter 14)
- Brachialis (chapter 28)
- Supinator (chapter 25)
- Triceps brachii (chapter 19)
- Supraspinatus (chapter 13)
- Trapezius (upper portion – chapter 10)
- Coracobrachialis (chapter 22)

Conclusion

Trigger points in the brachialis (chapter 28), supinator (chapter 25), triceps brachii (chapter 19), supraspinatus (chapter 13), trapezius (upper portion – chapter 10), and coracobrachialis (chapter 22) usually develop concurrently or within a few weeks' time of biceps trigger points, so you should also search for trigger points in those muscles. The same is true for the deltoid muscle (front portion), but since trigger points in that muscle don't directly cause elbow, lower arm, wrist, or hand pain, they are not addressed in this book. See the Resources section for books and other resources for self-treatment of muscles not covered in this book.

For books that contain a list of several other conditions that your medical health care provider may want to consider, see the Resources list.

Chapter 24

Hand Extensors;
Brachioradialis;
Finger Extensors

The use of computers has caused a huge increase in the number of patients with referred pain from trigger points in the forearm muscles. Often patients will complain of pain over the outside of the elbow or the back of the wrist, and may have been diagnosed with tennis elbow, tendinitis, or carpal tunnel syndrome. They are often given a brace to wear, which may afford some amount of relief but does not solve the trigger point–caused problem. See chapters 3 and 4 for additional information about tennis elbow, carpal tunnel syndrome, and other conditions.

Usually trigger points will form in more than one of the hand extensors or finger extensors, or the brachioradialis, and the self-help treatment is the same, so I have put them in one chapter.

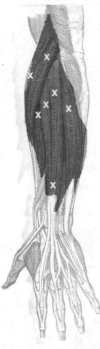

Back of forearm

Common Symptoms

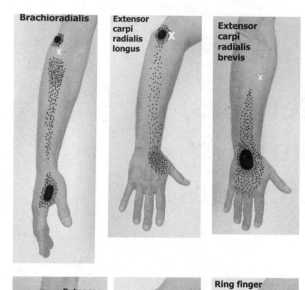

Brachioradialis

Extensor carpi radialis longus

Extensor carpi radialis brevis

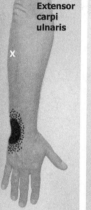

Extensor carpi ulnaris

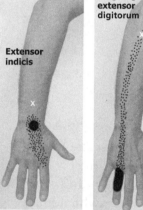

Extensor indicis

Ring finger extensor digitorum

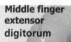

Middle finger extensor digitorum

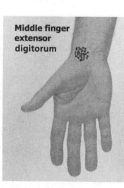

Middle finger extensor digitorum

- See the pictures for the various pain referral patterns, and consider that it is likely that more than one of these muscles is involved, causing a composite pain pattern rather than one of these individual patterns.

- With the hand extensors and brachioradialis muscles, pain is likely to first appear on the outside of the elbow, and then spread to the wrist and hand.

- Trigger points in finger extensors will cause finger stiffness, pain into the back of your forearm, hand, and fingers, and possibly into the elbow area, and arthritis-like pain in your finger joints.

- You will probably experience pain when shaking hands, turning a doorknob, using a screwdriver, or making any similar motions. The pain may be enough to wake you at night.

- You will probably experience a weakness of grip that causes you to unexpectedly drop items or spill when pouring or drinking (the larger the item, the more severe the problem).

- You will likely experience a loss of coordination and increased muscle fatigability while performing repetitive movements.

- Entrapment of the radial nerve may cause weakness of your backside forearm muscles, and/or numbness and tingling over the back of your hand.

Possible Causes and Perpetuators

- Gripping an object forcefully and repetitively; the larger the item, the more severe the problem. Examples are writing, weeding, shaking hands, using tools, ironing, throwing a Frisbee, scraping ice off a windshield, using a computer (especially the mouse arm,) waxing a car, giving a massage, using an adding machine, kayaking, and playing a violin or guitar.

- The extensor carpi ulnaris is more likely to develop trigger points after trauma, such as a broken arm, or after surgery or trauma in the shoulder joint or elbow.

- The finger extensors are likely to develop trigger points from repetitive finger movements such as playing the piano, carpentry, mechanical repairs, and playing with finger beads or rubber bands.

- Referral from trigger points in the scalene muscles can cause trigger points to form in the extensors carpi radialis or ulnaris, or extensor digitorum (ring and middle finger extensors).

- Referral from trigger points in the supraspinatus can cause trigger points to form in the extensor carpi radialis.

- Referral from trigger points in the serratus posterior superior can cause trigger points to form in the extensor carpi ulnaris.

- Trigger points in the supinator and brachioradialis usually form concurrently.

Helpful Hints

Avoid motions that require twisting your forearm and/or grasping repeatedly over long periods. Learn to alternate hands; for example, learn to use your computer mouse with both hands. Get a keyboard that is ergonomically correct.

A wrist brace can be worn temporarily until trigger points are relieved, but should not be considered a long-term solution. If you tend to curl your fist up under your chin in bed, prevent this by making a soft splint. Use an ACE bandage to strap a rolled towel over your forearm, wrist, and palm.

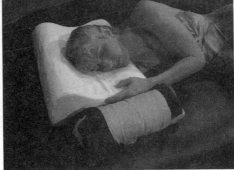

Muscle pain on the outside of the elbow is usually labeled "tennis elbow." The trigger points that cause pain in that area are likely to develop in the following order: (1) supinator, (2) brachioradialis, (3) extensor carpi radialis longus, (4) extensor digitorum, (5) triceps brachii, (6) anconeus, and (7) the biceps brachii and brachialis together (see below for chapter numbers). See chapter 3 for more information on tennis elbow.

Self-Help Techniques

Applying Pressure

Hand and Finger Extensors Pressure

Place your forearm across your lap. If you have large breasts, you may need to rest your arm on a table in front of you. Using your other elbow, apply pressure to the muscles on the outside and back of the forearm. Push the muscle on the thumb side (the brachioradialis) out of the way toward your trunk to also access the extensor carpi radialis longus underneath it, which is a very important muscle to work on.

Alternatively, use a golf ball cradled in the palm of your hand. Rotate the elbow of that hand out in front of you so that you don't stress the forearm muscles in the arm you are using to treat the affected arm, and press the golf ball into tender spots.

Then to get points your elbow can't reach, with your forearm on a flat surface and your palm face up, use the opposite hand to help press your forearm onto the golf ball. Be careful not to hurt your back if you do this last part.

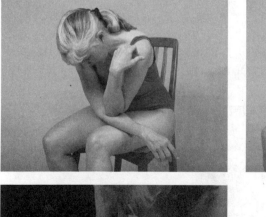
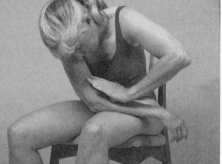
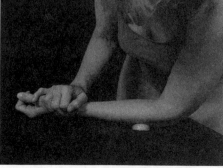

Stretches

Finger Extensor Stretch

To stretch the finger extensors, put your forearm in front of your lower chest, with your elbow bent at about 90 degrees, palm up, and your hand bent upward at the wrist and in a fist. Use your opposite hand to assist in a gentle stretch.

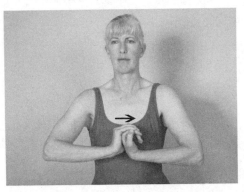

Artisan's Stretch

Put your hands out in front of you, palms out and fingers spread. At the same time as you slowly rotate your hands to palms up, start making a fist, starting with your little finger. By the time your hand is fully rotated, the fist is complete and you also bend at your wrist.

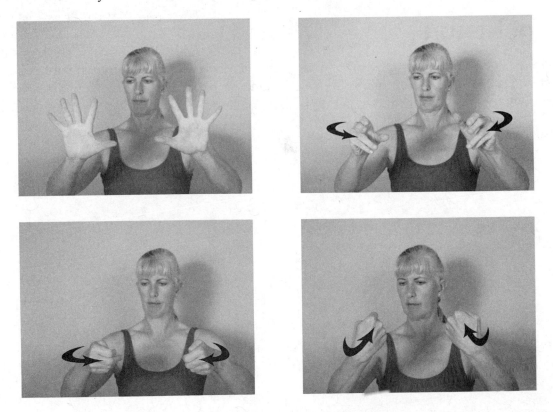

Finger Flutter Exercise

See chapter 27 for this exercise.

Also See

- Triceps brachii, anconeus (chapter 19)
- Biceps brachii (chapter 23)
- Supinator (chapter 25)
- Brachialis (chapter 28)
- Scalenes (chapter 20)
- Serratus posterior superior (chapter 15)
- Supraspinatus (chapter 13)
- Brachioradialis (chapter 24)
- Extensor carpi radialis longus (chapter 24)
- Extensor digitorum (chapter 24)

Conclusion

You may need to see a chiropractor or osteopathic physician to check for volar subluxation of the wrist bones or distal radioulnar joint dysfunction. For books that contain a list of several other conditions that your medical health care provider may want to consider, see the Resources list.

Chapter 25

Supinator

Pain from trigger points in the supinator is frequently diagnosed as tennis elbow, though there is usually a lack of recognition by many practitioners that trigger points are the causative factor. The hand and finger extensors are commonly also involved. Surgery is probably unnecessary, so try the trigger point self-help techniques first.

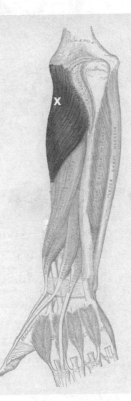

Back of forearm

Common Symptoms

- Trigger points refer aching pain to the outside of the elbow and web of the thumb, and possibly to the back of the forearm. There might be tenderness with tapping on the outside of the elbow.

- Pain probably continues even after the aggravating activity is stopped.

- Trigger points may possibly cause entrapment of the radial nerve, which leads to weakness with opening your hand and uncomfortable sensations on the back of your wrist and forearm.

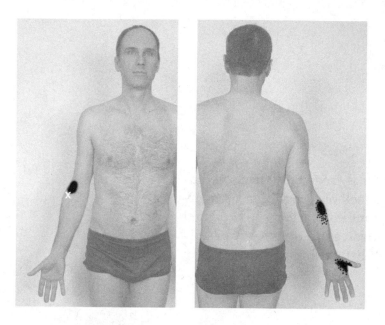

Possible Causes and Perpetuators

- Carrying a heavy briefcase with the arm straight, or hoisting a briefcase onto a desk into the ready-to-open position

- Placing a sudden strain on the muscle

- Doing activities such as walking a dog on a leash, wringing clothes, ironing, turning stiff doorknobs, unscrewing a tight jar lid, shaking hands repetitively, washing walls, raking leaves, waxing a car, giving massages, and playing tennis, especially with the arm held straight

Helpful Hints

Carry packages with your palms faceup. Get a briefcase with a shoulder strap that can be worn diagonally across your torso rather than carrying it hanging from one hand. Lift it onto a table with both hands rather than swinging it up with one hand.

If you play tennis, keep your elbow slightly bent, and the head of the racquet slightly up. A lighter racquet and a smaller handle will also be helpful. Don't play every day, in order to give your muscles a chance to recuperate.

When shaking hands try to alternate hands, and offer your palm faceup. Train your dog not to pull on the leash, or switch hands. Get a head halter so the dog is not able to pull so much. Don't rake leaves.

An elastic support with a hole for the point of the elbow may be worn during activities that aggravate the supinator, but this should only be worn for short periods due to reduced circulation to the muscles.

Self-Help Techniques

Applying Pressure

Supinator Pressure

Place your forearm across your lap with your palm up (if you have large breasts, you may need to try resting your arm on a table in front of you). Using your opposite elbow, apply pressure to the muscles on the *upper third front of the forearm, particularly close to the elbow crease and from the middle to the outside of the forearm.*

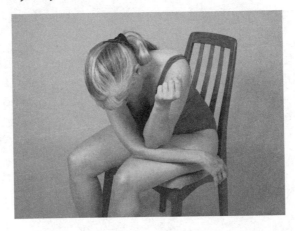

Alternatively, use a golf ball cradled in the palm of your hand, rotate the elbow of that hand out in front of you so you don't stress the forearm muscles in the arm you are *using* to treat the affected arm, and press the golf ball into tender spots.

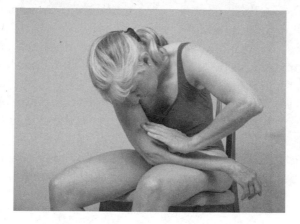

Also See

- Triceps brachii (chapter 19)
- Hand extensors, brachioradialis, finger extensors (chapter 24)
- Brachialis (chapter 28)
- Biceps brachii (chapter 23)
- Palmaris longus (chapter 26)

Conclusion

Trigger points are also often found concurrently in the triceps brachii (chapter 19) and finger extensors and brachioradialis (chapter 24) muscles, so you will want to search those for trigger points too. The brachialis (chapter 28), biceps brachii (chapter 23), and sometimes the palmaris longus (chapter 26) muscles may also get involved.

You may need to see a chiropractor or osteopathic physician for evaluation of articular dysfunction of the distal radioulnar joint. For books that contain a list of several other conditions that your medical health care provider may want to consider, see the Resources list.

Chapter 26

Palmaris Longus

The palmaris longus may be absent or variable in its location along the forearm. Due to the wrist and hand pain and tenderness associated with trigger points in the palmaris longus muscle, symptoms may be mistaken for carpal tunnel syndrome. In this case, trigger point self-help will relieve the symptoms. However, because of the variable location of this muscle, if it extends under the carpel ligament, it may cause *true* carpal tunnel syndrome. Trigger points in the muscle would increase tension in the tendon and would aggravate carpal tunnel symptoms, and self-help would likely only partially relieve symptoms.

In advanced cases, this muscle and its action on cutaneous tissue in the palm are a factor in the development of the nodules, fibrous bands, and pain of Dupuytren's contracture. See chapter 4 for a discussion of this condition.

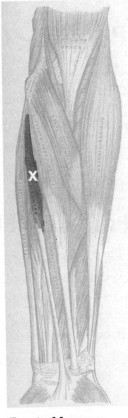

Front of forearm

Common Symptoms

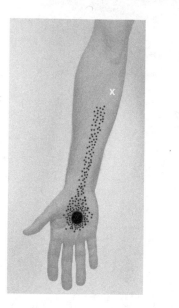

- Trigger points refer pain that is felt in the palm and possibly in the front of the forearm, and feels superficial and similar to being pricked with a needle.

- You probably have difficulty in handling tools due to tenderness in your palm.

- Variable palmaris longus muscle configurations and attachments may cause pain in the back of the lower arm, compression neuropathy, or a "dead feeling" in the forearms.

- In advanced cases of Dupuytren's contracture, the palm is contracted and you would be unable to lay your hand flat on a surface.

Possible Causes and Perpetuators

- Referred pain from the middle head of the triceps near the elbow, causing satellite trigger points in the palmaris longus muscle

- Experiencing a direct trauma, such as falling on your outstretched hand

- Holding tools and racquets improperly, allowing them to dig forcibly into your palm

Helpful Hints

Don't use any tool or sports equipment that continues to dig into the palm.

Trigger point self-help techniques and acupuncture, especially plum blossom technique over the nodules and needles inserted into the palmaris longus and other hand and finger flexors (chapter 27), may possibly help stop the progression of Dupuytren's contracture. See chapter 4 for more information.

Self-Help Techniques

Applying Pressure

Palmaris Longus Pressure

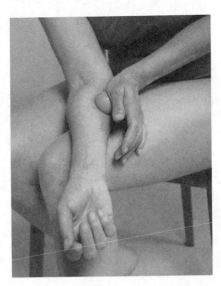

Place your forearm across your lap (if you have large breasts, you may need to try resting your arm on a table in front of you). Using your other elbow, apply pressure to the muscles on the front of the forearm, particularly close to the elbow crease. Alternatively, use a golf ball cradled in the palm of your hand, rotate the elbow of that side out in front of you so you don't stress the forearm muscles in the arm you are using to treat the affected arm, and press the golf ball into tender spots.

Stretches

Anterior Forearm Stretch

See chapter 27 for this stretch.

Also See

- Hand and finger flexors (chapter 27)

Conclusion

Be sure to treat the triceps muscle first, since it will refer pain to the palmaris longus area and perpetuate trigger points.

Chapter 27

Hand and Finger Flexors
(Flexor Carpi Radialis and Ulnaris, Flexores Digitorum Superficialis and Profundus, Flexor Pollicis Longus, and Pronator Teres)

Trigger points in the hand and finger flexors are common, though not as common as in the hand and finger extensors. It is a good idea to treat both sides of the forearm.

Often trigger points in the hand and finger flexors develop as satellite trigger points, so it is important to work on the primary trigger points first; see below for the list of muscles to check.

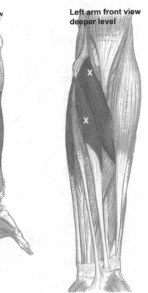

Left arm front view

Left arm front view
deeper level

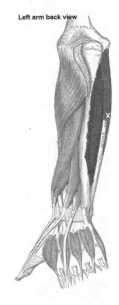

Left arm back view

Common Symptoms

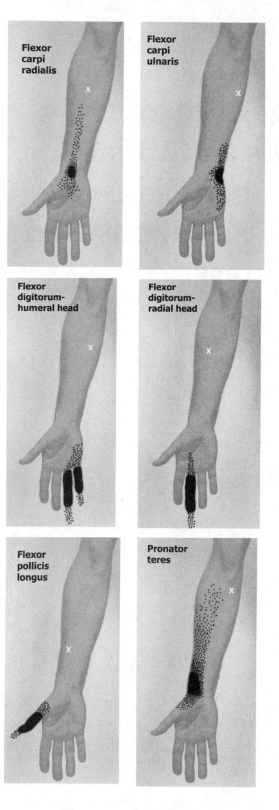

- Pain refers in various patterns over the front of the forearm, the front of the wrist, the palm, and the fingers and thumb. See the pictures for the various pain referral patterns.

- Pain can feel as if it projects off the ends of the thumb and fingers, like a "bolt of lightening."

- You may experience finger stiffness and painful cramping, difficulty in using scissors, one-handed garden clippers, or tin shears, or difficulty putting curlers, bobby pins, or clips in your hair. You may experience an inability to cup your hand while your palm is face up, as when brushing something off of a counter into your cupped hand.

- Symptoms are aggravated by stress, cold drafts, and loud noises.

- "Trigger finger," where your finger gets "stuck" in the fist-closed position, is caused by a constriction of a tendon in the palm, about one thumb's width above the crease between your palm and the affected finger.

- Entrapment of the ulnar nerve at your elbow can cause uncomfortable sensations, burning pain, numbness, and loss of sensation in your fourth and fifth fingers, and may lead to clumsiness and grip weakness.

Possible Causes and Perpetuators

- Repetitive gripping of small-handled tools, gripping a steering wheel or ski poles too firmly, giving massages, or punching holes with a one-handed hole punch repetitively, as when punching tickets or receipts at events or store entrances.

- Kayaking or canoeing.

- Weeding a garden can cause trigger points to form in the flexor pollicis longus muscle.

- Receiving a fracture at the wrist or elbow can cause trigger points to form in the pronator teres muscle.

- The cause of trigger finger is unclear, but it may possibly be pressing something relatively pointy repeatedly into the palm.

Helpful Hints

Avoid pressing anything into your palm repeatedly. When using small-handled tools, rest and stretch frequently, and change activities frequently if possible. If using a one-handed hole punch, switch hands often and trade off frequently with other personnel if possible.

Learn to relax your grip when steering or skiing, and hold onto the sides of the steering wheel. If you are rowing with an oar, uncurl your fingers as the oar sweeps back. When kayaking, "feathering" your paddle may help. Stretch your fingers frequently. Racquets should be held slightly up rather than tilted down.

Keep your hand and forearm supported when sitting.

"Trigger finger" may be relieved either by needling (by acupuncture or hypodermic needle) or possibly by applying pressure to a tender spot in the palm fairly close to the affected finger, about opposite the knuckle when you look at the hand from the side.

Self-Help Techniques

Applying Pressure

Hand and Finger Flexors Pressure

Place your forearm across your lap with your palm face up. If you have large breasts, you may need to try resting your arm on a table in front of you. Using your other elbow, apply pressure to the muscles on the front upper two-thirds of the forearm.

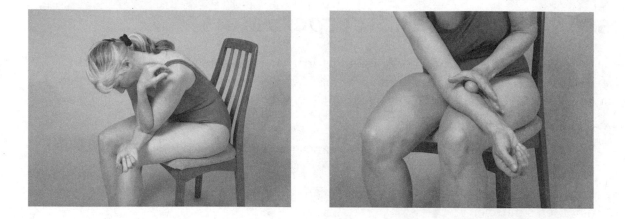

Alternatively, use a golf ball cradled in the palm of your hand and press the golf ball into tender spots.

Stretches

Perform these stretches frequently.

Anterior Forearm Stretch

With your arms at your sides, find a surface about the height of your palm. Point the fingers backward, and keeping your arm straight, press the palm into the surface, so you are getting a stretch on the front of the forearm.

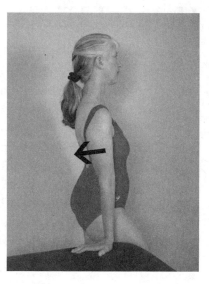

Finger Extension Stretch

Support your elbow on the side to be stretched. Using the palm of the opposite side, gently stretch your fingers back until you feel a stretch in your fingers, palm, and forearm.

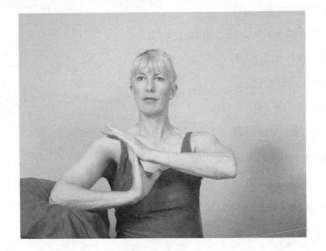

Finger Flutter

Put your arms at your sides and shake your hands, keeping your wrist and fingers loose so your lower arm gets a benefit too.

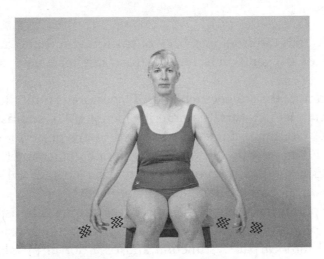

Artisan's Stretch

See chapter 24 for this stretch.

Interossei Stretch

See chapter 30 for this stretch

Also See

- Scalenes (chapter 20)
- Pectoralis minor (chapter 21)
- Pectoralis major and subclavius (chapter 11)
- Serratus anterior (chapter 12)
- Supraspinatus (chapter 13)
- Infraspinatus (chapter 14)
- Latissimus dorsi (chapter 17)
- Serratus posterior superior (chapter 15)
- Triceps brachii (chapter 19)
- Hand extensors and brachioradialis (chapter 24)
- Palmaris longus (chapter 26)
- Adductor pollicis and opponens pollicis (chapter 29)

Conclusion

It is a good idea to work both the front and back of the forearm (hand and finger extensors – chapter 24), since relief of trigger points on the front can reactivate trigger points on the backside.

You may also need to treat the scalenes (chapter 20), pectoralis minor (chapter 21), pectoralis major and subclavius (chapter 11), serratus anterior (chapter 12), supraspinatus (chapter 13), infraspinatus (chapter 14), latissimus dorsi (chapter 17), serratus posterior superior (chapter 15), triceps brachii (chapter 19), hand extensors and brachioradialis (chapter 24), palmaris longus (chapter 26), and/or adductor pollicis and opponens pollicis (chapter 29), since they can cause satellite trigger points to develop in the hand and finger flexors.

Referral from trigger points in the hand and finger flexors may get misdiagnosed as thoracic outlet syndrome (see chapter 3). You may need to see a chiropractor or osteopathic physician to be evaluated for a distal radiocarpal dysfunction and/or a dorsal misalignment of the wrist bones. For books that contain a list of several other conditions that your medical health care provider may want to consider, see the Resources list.

Chapter 28

Brachialis

Trigger points in the brachialis muscle are fairly common, and may be misdiagnosed as either as arthritis or some kind of problem with the wrist, due to its primary referral pattern.

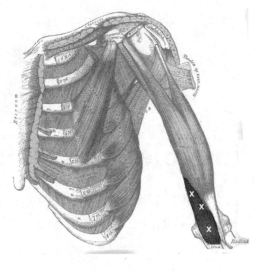

View of front of body

Common Symptoms

- Trigger points refer pain or tenderness around the base of the thumb, and the thumb pad. Some pain may be present at the crease opposite the elbow, and perhaps over the front of the upper arm.

- You may experience a loss of sensation, tingling, and numbness on the back side of the thumb if the radial nerve is entrapped by trigger points in the brachialis.

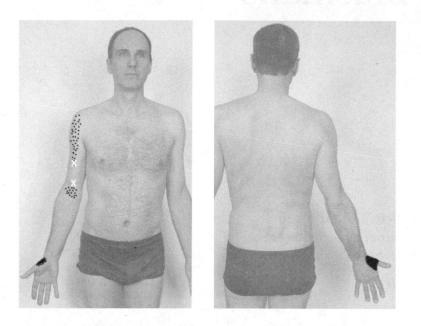

Possible Causes and Perpetuators

- Lifting heavy items, holding a power tool, or carrying groceries
- Playing a guitar or violin
- Ironing meticulously
- Using crutches
- Trigger points in the supinator (chapter 25) can cause satellite trigger points in the brachialis and biceps muscles.

Helpful Hints

Avoid lifting heavy items, and when you lift lighter items, keep your palms faceup. Get a purse with a long strap that can be worn diagonally across your torso rather than carrying your purse in your hand.

When playing an instrument, stretch your arm out whenever possible. Use a headset or speaker phone when talking on the phone, or use the opposite arm to hold a phone to your ear.

At night, be sure not to draw your arm tightly into your body. Instead, try to keep the elbow out from the body. You may try putting a pillow in the crook of your elbow to help with this.

Self-Help Techniques

Applying Pressure

Brachialis Pressure

Using your opposite hand, hook your thumb around the inside of your upper arm, and use your finger to move the biceps toward your thumb and torso while at the same time pressing into the muscle underneath. The area extends from about the middle of the upper arm, down almost to the elbow crease.

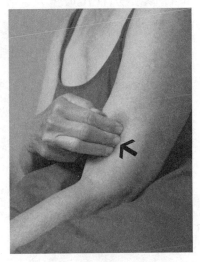

Stretches

Brachialis Stretch

While supporting your upper arm just above the elbow on a chair or couch arm and with the palm faceup, use the opposite hand to push down gently on the inside of the wrist.

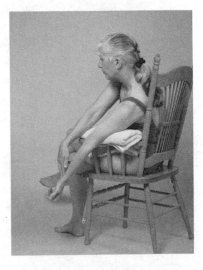

Also See

- Biceps brachii (chapter 23)
- Brachioradialis (chapter 24)
- Supinator (chapter 25)
- Adductor pollicis and opponens pollicis (chapter 29)

Conclusion

For books that contain a list of several other conditions that your medical health care provider may want to consider, see the Resources list.

Chapter 29

Adductor Pollicis;
Opponens Pollicis

Referred pain from trigger points in the adductor and opponens
pollicis muscles can be erroneously attributed to a joint problem,
and patients will frequently self-diagnose with "arthritis." These
are relatively common trigger points.

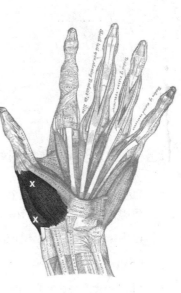

Common Symptoms

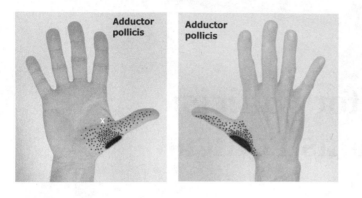

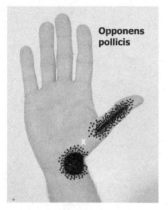

- Trigger points refer aching pain over your thumb pad, into your thumb, and over part of your wrist.

- You may experience weakness and difficulty with any fine motor movements that require your thumb to grasp, such as sewing, buttoning a shirt, writing, or holding onto items.

- "Trigger thumb," where the thumb locks in the closed position, can be caused by a tender spot in or near one of the forearm flexor tendons located under the thumb pad or in the web between the thumb and first finger

Possible Causes and Perpetuators

- Using fine motor movements to do activities such as weeding a garden (particularly with difficult-to-pull weeds), sewing, crocheting, knitting, or handwriting

- Using small paint brushes for artwork

- Giving massages

- Having residual pain from a fracture

Helpful Hints

Take frequent breaks when sewing, crocheting, knitting, writing, and painting. When weeding, loosen the dirt with a spade first, weed only for short periods, and alternate hands.

Self-Help Techniques

Applying Pressure

Adductor and Opponens Pollicis Pressure

If your opposite thumb is not also affected, you may use that thumb to apply pressure all over and around the thumb pad on the affected side. If both thumbs are affected, use the eraser on the end of a pencil to apply pressure. Some massage stores sell pressure devices that are easily held in the palm of the hand. Just be sure you use a pressure tip that is not much bigger than the eraser on the top of a pencil, or you will not get enough focused pressure for the trigger points.

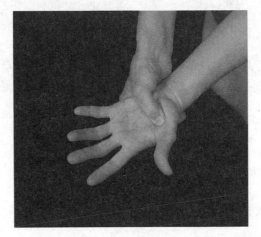

Stretches

Adductor Pollicis Stretch

Place both hands on a surface in front of you, with index finger to index finger and thumb to thumb, with the thumbs pointed back toward you and the palms flat on the surface. You may also do this in warm water.

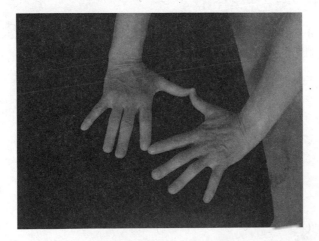

Opponens Pollicis Stretch

With your palm faceup, use your opposite hand to reach underneath the hand you are treating, and pull down gently on the thumb.

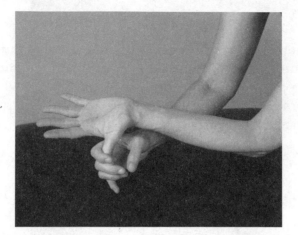

Artisan's Stretch

See chapter 24 for this stretch.

Finger Flutter Exercise

See chapter 27 for this exercise.

Interossei Stretch

See chapter 30 for this stretch

Anterior Forearm Stretch

See chapter 27 for this stretch.

Also See

- Scalenes (chapter 20)
- Brachialis (chapter 28)
- Supinator (chapter 25)
- Hand extensors, Brachioradialis, and Finger extensors (extensor carpi radialis longus) (chapter 24)
- Hand interossei (chapter 30)

Conclusion

Also consider trigger points in the scalenes (chapter 20), brachialis (chapter 28), supinator (chapter 25), and hand extensors (extensor carpi radialis longus) and brachioradialis (chapter 24) muscles, since they can also refer pain to this area, and should be treated prior to the thumb muscles. Active trigger points are almost always also found in the hand interosseous muscles (chapter 30) between the thumb and first finger.

You may need to see a chiropractor or osteopathic physician to be evaluated for misalignments of a metacarpal or carpal bone, especially at the thumb carpometacarpal joint. For books that contain a list of several other conditions that your medical health care provider may want to consider, see the Resources list.

Chapter 30

Hand Interossei; Abductor Digiti Minimi

People with interosseous trigger points frequently self-diagnose as having arthritis, because of referred pain around the finger joints. Interestingly, inactivating trigger points in the interosseous muscles and resolving any applicable perpetuating factors may actually help delay or stop the progression of some types of osteoarthritis.

Trigger points in the interosseous muscles may possibly contribute to the formation of Heberden's nodes, hard bumps (initially tender) about the size of a pea on one side of the joint closest to the fingertip; see chapter 4 for more information.

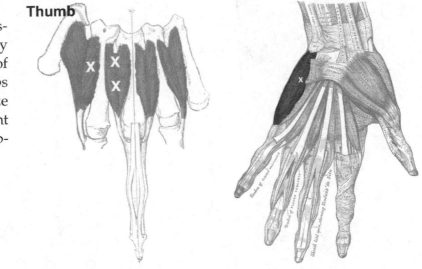

Back of hand

Back of hand

Common Symptoms

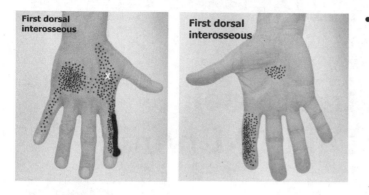

First dorsal interosseous

First dorsal interosseous

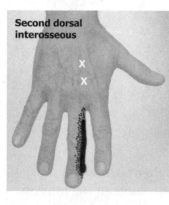

Second dorsal interosseous

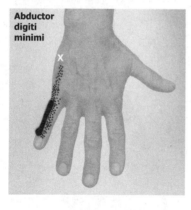

Abductor digiti minimi

- Trigger points refer pain down one or more fingers and the backside and palm of the hand. The pain is usually worse on one side of the joint closest to the fingertip. Note that the pictures show examples of referral patterns, but trigger points can develop in any of these small muscles and cause subsequent referral to either side of any finger.

- You may experience difficulty in bringing your fingers together or making a fist, or finger stiffness that interferes with fine motor movements such as buttoning, writing, and grasping objects.

- An interosseous muscle may entrap a finger's nerve, causing superficial numbness on one side of your finger.

Possible Causes and Perpetuators

- Grasping repetitively with your fingers pinched together—for example, pulling weeds, gripping golf clubs tightly, giving massages, or using small tools, paint-brushes, and needles

Helpful Hints

Learn not to grasp items tightly, and take frequent breaks. Limit the amount of time for any given activity.

If you have Heberden's nodes, look for trigger points in the interosseous muscles. Once the trigger points are inactivated, tenderness should disappear immediately, and over time the node itself will probably disappear.

Self-Help Techniques

Applying Pressure

Interossei Pressure

Buy pencil erasers that fit on the end of a pencil. Using the tip of the eraser, press in between the bones of the hand on both the back side and the palm side.

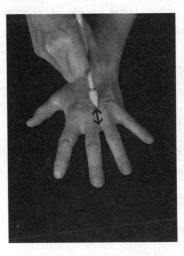
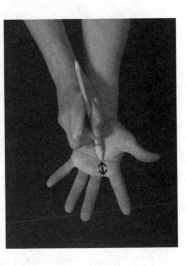

Abductor Digiti Minimi Pressure

Use your opposite thumb to work on the outside edge of the hand, or pinch the muscle in between your opposite thumb and fingers.

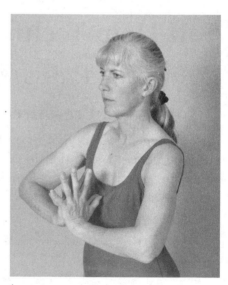

Stretches

Interosseous Stretch

With your forearms in front of your chest, palm to palm and fingers to fingers, separate your fingers and press your palms against each other with the fingers pointed upward, so your fingers and the front of your forearms are getting a good stretch.

Adductor Pollicis Stretch

See chapter 29 for this stretch.

Artisan's Stretch

See chapter 24 for this stretch.

Finger Flutter Exercise

See chapter 27 for this exercise.

Anterior Forearm Stretch

See chapter 27 for this stretch.

Also See

- Adductor pollicis and opponens pollicis (chapter 29)
- Hand and finger flexors (chapter 27)
- Hand extensors and brachioradialis (chapter 24)
- Latissimus dorsi (chapter 17)
- Pectoralis major (chapter 11)
- Pectoralis minor (chapter 21)
- Scalenes (chapter 20)
- Triceps brachii (chapter 19)

Conclusion

Also consider trigger points in the adductor pollicis and opponens pollicis (chapter 29), hand and finger flexors (chapter 27), hand extensors and brachioradialis (chapter 24), latissimus dorsi (chapter 17), pectoralis major (chapter 11), pectoralis minor (chapter 21), scalenes (chapter 20), and triceps brachii (chapter 19) muscles.

You may need to see a chiropractor or osteopathic physician to be evaluated for misalignment of bones in the hand. For books that contain a list of several other conditions that your medical health care provider may want to consider, see the Resources list.

Resources

Books

These books contain lists of several other conditions that your medical health care provider may want to consider:

DeLaune, Valerie. 2004. *Pain Relief with Trigger Point Self-Help.* Juneau, AK: Alaskan Natural Care, Inc.

Simons, D. G., J. G. Travell, and L. S. Simons. 1999. *Myofascial Pain and Dysfunction: The Trigger Point Manual.* Vol. 1, *The Upper Half of the Body,* 2nd ed. Baltimore, MD: Lippincott Williams & Wilkins.

Travell, J. G., and D. G. Simons. 1983. *Myofascial Pain and Dysfunction: The Trigger Point Manual,* 1st ed. Baltimore, MD: Lippincott Williams & Wilkins.

Travell, J. G., and D. G. Simons. 1999. *Myofascial Pain and Dysfunction: The Trigger Point Manual,* 2nd ed. Baltimore, MD: Lippincott Williams & Wilkins.

Other Resources

New Harbinger Publications. New Harbinger publishes books on a variety of self-help topics that you may find helpful. 800-748-6273. newharbinger.com.

The Pressure Positive Company. This company sells self-pressure devices and massage tools. Its website has an information center with articles and links to other helpful sites. 800-603-5107. pressurepositive.com.

Superfeet. This company sells noncorrective footbeds, and its website can help you locate a dealer who can make Superfeet custom footbeds for you. 800-634-6618. superfeet.com.

TriggerPointRelief.com. Author's website with additional resources, articles, and links to helpful sites.

References

Audette, J. F., F. Wang, and H. Smith. 2004. Bilateral activation of motor unit potentials with uni-lateral needle stimulation of active myofascial trigger points. *American Journal of Physical Medicine and Rehabilitation* 83 (5):368–74.

Balch, J. F., and P. A. Balch. 2000. *Prescription for Nutritional Healing: A Practical A–Z Reference to Drug-Free Remedies Using Vitamins, Minerals, Herbs, and Food Supplements.* New York: Avery.

Borg-Stein, J., and D. G. Simons. 2002. Myofascial pain. *Archives of Physical Medicine and Rehabilitation* 83 (Suppl 1):S40–47.

Chen Q., S. Bensamoun, J. R. Basford, J. M. Thompson, and K. N. An. 2007. Identification of myo-fascial taut bands with magnetic resonance elastography. *Archives of Physical Medicine and Rehabilitation* 88:1658–1661.

Edwards, J., and N. Knowles. 2003. Superficial dry needling and active stretching in the treat-ment of myofascial pain: A randomised controlled trial. *Acupuncture in Medicine* 21 (3):80–86.

Heath, K. M., and E. P. Elovic. Vitamin D deficiency: Implications in the rehabilitation setting. *American Journal of Physical Medicine and Rehabilitation* 85:916–923.

Issbener, U., P. Reeh, and K. Steen. 1996. Pain due to tissue acidosis: A mechanism for inflamma-tory and ischemic myalgia? *Neuroscience Letters* 208 (1996):191–194.

Latremoliere, A., and C. J. Woolf. 2009. Central sensitization: A generator of pain hypersensitivity by central neural plasticity. *The Journal of Pain* 10 (9):895–926.

Marcus, D. A., L. Scharff, S. Mercer, and D. C. Turk. 1999. Musculoskeletal abnormalities in chronic headache: A controlled comparison of headache diagnostic groups. *Headache: The Journal of Head and Face Pain* 39 (1):21–27.

Niddam, D. M. 2009. Brain manifestation and modulation of pain from myofascial trigger points. *Current Pain and Headache Reports* 13:370–375.

Partanen, J., T. A. Ojala, and J. P. A. Arokoski. 2009. Myofascial syndrome and pain: A neurophysiologic approach. *Pathophysiology*, doi:10.10266/j.pathophus.2009.05.001.

Shah, J. P., J. V. Danoff, M. J. Desai, S. Parikh, L. Y. Nakamura, T. M. Phillips, and L. H. Gerber. 2008. Biochemicals associated with pain and inflammation are elevated in sites near to and remote from active myofascial trigger points. *Archives of Physical Medicine and Rehabilitation* 89:16–23.

Simons, D. G. 2003. Enigmatic trigger points often cause enigmatic musculoskeletal pain. Presentation at the STAR Symposium, Columbus, Ohio, May 22. Available at http://ergonom ics.osu.edu/pdfs/2003%20STAR%20Symposium/Simons%20Trigger.pdf.

———. 2004. Review of enigmatic MTrPs as a common cause of enigmatic musculoskeletal pain and dysfunction. *Journal of Electromyography and Kinesiology* 14 (1):95–107.

Simons, D. G., J. G. Travell, and L. S. Simons. 1999. *Myofascial Pain and Dysfunction: The Trigger Point Manual*. Vol. 1, *The Upper Half of the Body*, 2nd ed. Baltimore, MD: Lippincott Williams & Wilkins.

Travell, J. G., and D. G. Simons. 1983. *Myofascial Pain and Dysfunction: The Trigger Point Manual*. Baltimore, MD: Lippincott Williams & Wilkins.

———. 1992. *Myofascial Pain and Dysfunction: The Trigger Point Manual*. Vol. 2, *The Lower Extremities*. Baltimore, MD: Lippincott Williams & Wilkins.

Valerie DeLaune, LAc, is a licensed acupuncturist and certified neuromuscular therapist. She holds a master's degree in acupuncture from the Northwest Institute of Acupuncture and Oriental Medicine. She has authored books and articles on trigger points, acupuncture, health, and environmental topics. DeLaune resides in Anchorage, AK. www.triggerpointrelief.com

Foreword writer **Renee Gladieux Principe, NCTMB,** is a retired US Army Captain, practicing massage therapist, and director of sales for The Pressure Positive Company, a family-owned, massage tool manufacturing company. She lives in Gilbertsville, PA.

Index

pollicis muscle, 178; in anconeus muscle, 132; in biceps brachii muscle, 150; in brachialis muscle, 174; in brachioradialis muscle, 154; in coracobrachialis muscle, 146; in finger extensors, 154; in finger flexors, 168; in hand extensors, 154; in hand flexors, 168; in hand interossei, 184; in infraspinatus muscle, 106; in latissimus dorsi muscle, 122; in opponens pollicis muscle, 178; in palmaris longus muscle, 164; in pectoralis major muscle, 88; in pectoralis minor muscle, 142; in scalene muscles, 136; in serratus anterior muscle, 96; in serratus posterior superior muscle, 112; in subclavius muscle, 89; in subscapularis muscle, 117; in supinator muscle, 160; in supraspinatus muscle, 102; in teres major muscle, 128; in trapezius muscle, 80–81; in triceps brachii muscle, 132

synapses, 8

T

TDP heating lamp, 116
telephone headsets, 33, 137, 175
tendinitis, 110, 153
tennis elbow, 21–22, 153, 156, 159
tension, noticing, 55
teres major muscle, 127–130; applying pressure to, 129; causes/perpetuators of trigger points in, 128; helpful hints related to, 128; illustration of, 127; self-help techniques, 129; stretching, 129; symptoms of trigger points in, 128
thoracic outlet syndrome (TOS), 22–23, 89, 127, 135
thrower's elbow, 22
thyroid function, 58–59
tobacco use, 51
trapezius muscle, 79–86; applying pressure to, 82–84; causes/perpetuators of trigger points in, 81; helpful hints related to, 82; illustration of, 79; proper posture and, 86;

self-help techniques, 82–86; stretching, 85; symptoms of trigger points in, 80–81
traumatic injuries, 21
Travell, Janet, ix–x, 17, 29
treatment: doctor visits and, 18; importance of prompt, 16–17; time required for, 17–18. *See also* self-treatments
triceps brachii muscle, 131–134; applying pressure to, 133; causes/perpetuators of trigger points in, 133; helpful hints related to, 133; illustration of, 131; self-help techniques, 133–134; stretching, 134; symptoms of trigger points in, 132
trigger finger/thumb, 27, 168, 178
trigger point therapy: self-treatment with, 65–68; time required for, 17–18; why it works, 16–17
Trigger Point Therapy for Headaches & Migraines (DeLaune), 79
trigger points: active vs. latent, 10; biochemical measures of, 11; body mechanics and, 31–39; characteristics of, 7–11; dietary factors and, 41–52; emotional factors and, 53–55; formation of, 13; injuries and, 24, 27, 36–37; locating within muscles, 67; organ dysfunction/disease and, 58–60; perpetuating factors for, 29–61; pH acidity and, 11; primary and satellite, 10–11; problems from untreated, 11–13; referred pain from, 1, 8–9, 74; self-treatment guidelines, 65–68; sleep problems and, 55–56; symptoms of, 7–10; treating, 16–18
TriggerPointRelief.com website, 190

U

upper trapezius muscle: common symptoms, 80; upper trapezius pinch, 84
urinary tract infections, 57

V

vegetarianism, 44

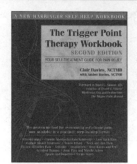
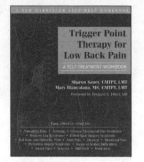
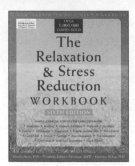
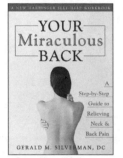
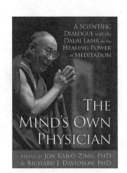